Essential Oils for Hormones

The Ultimate Beginners Guide to Improve Inflammation, Weight Gain, Sleep, Anxiety, Depression, and Other Hormonal Imbalance Symptoms

Elle Washington

professional advice. The content within this book has been derived from various sources. Please consult a licensed professional before attempting any techniques outlined in this book.

By reading this document, the reader agrees that under no circumstances is the author responsible for any losses, direct or indirect, that are incurred as a result of the use of the information contained within this document, including, but not limited to, errors, omissions, or inaccuracies.

Table of Contents

Introduction

Have you struggled with sleeplessness, anxiety, and depression? Do you find it almost impossible to drag yourself out of bed in the mornings or get to sleep in the evenings? How is your overall mental wellbeing? Do you struggle to wind down or relax? Do your thoughts race every time your head hits your pillow? How are you coping with the stress of life? These are all questions that you have probably thought about consistently. Maybe you haven't answered them because you are busy, or afraid, or in denial. Whatever the reason may be, you are here, reading this book. Asking yourself those questions can help you to use essential oils in a positive, transformative, and holistic way. Life can be overwhelming and chaotic and before you realize that you should start listening to your body, it is already screaming for help. However, it is never too late to take ownership of the predicament in which you find yourself. In this book, I will help you to understand your body and show you how you can use essential oils to alleviate the symptoms of hormonal imbalance.

Perhaps you don't struggle with depression and anxiety but, rather, find yourself experiencing a hormonal imbalance of a different kind, like digestive issues, lowered libido, or polycystic ovary syndrome (PCOS). The body produces many hormones and they all work together in perfect unison to make sure your body functions as it is supposed to. Each hormone plays an integral part in human survival. Not only that, but the *quantity* of the hormones produced is precise. In this way, it not only matters that each and every hormone must be present in the body, it matters that the quantities of these hormones must also be exact. Say, for instance, you get a fright and adrenaline (a hormone) starts pulsing through your body. Your heart beats faster, your pupils dilate, your hands begin to sweat, and you are ready to go into fight or flight mode. The body releases a specific amount of adrenaline into the bloodstream to prompt the correct and appropriate response to a stimulus. However, if your body were to release too much adrenaline, you could suffer serious, if not fatal, heart damage. While you shouldn't be too worried about scaring yourself to death—literally—the point of this analogy is to highlight the importance of balanced hormones. If one of these hormones is even slightly off-balance, it could prompt a series of negative reactions within the body. For example, having too much cortisol in your body could result in memory loss or anxiety. Having too little testosterone could lead to hair loss or lowered libido. Alternatively, having too much testosterone could lead to infertility or acne.

Think of it like a cake. People have been making cakes for hundreds of years and, while each cake is different and requires different ingredients, they all have a specific structure. Cakes consist of sugar, flour, baking powder, eggs, and milk. Yes, some cakes include apples and some use buttermilk instead of milk. Some cakes use brown sugar and others use whole-wheat flour. The different cakes available are kind of like the different humans that exist. Everyone has their own structure but the basic recipe stays the same. All healthy human bodies consist of the same *eggs, flour, sugar* structure that a cake does, except for humans, these ingredients are known as hormones. Similarly, when making a cake, if you put too many eggs in the batter, the cake will be stodgy and dense. If you put too much baking powder in the cake, it will fall flat and taste acidic. If your hormones are imbalanced, your body will react accordingly. Remember what famous physicist Isaac Newton said, *for every action, there is an equal and opposite reaction*. And it doesn't just end there. You still have to bake the cake. If you bake it at too high a temperature, the cake will burn, and if you bake it at too low a temperature, it will never cook. You can't expect to live a stressed life without ever taking care of your body and brain and have all of your hormones perfectly balanced. If you indulge in junk food and neglect your body's needs, or don't bring mindfulness into your life, your mind, body, and soul will suffer. Whether your hormonal imbalance has led to physical or mental symptoms, these manifestations can make living a full and healthy life rather challenging. Luckily for you, I will provide you with the necessary skills to approach your life holistically and healthily using essential oils and other useful practices.

Whatever your plight, you are here because you are probably suffering from something that you hope to cure or improve with essential oils. Maybe you have tried everything and are at your wit's end. Pharmaceuticals haven't worked, exercise has only incrementally improved your lifestyle, you have seen countless doctors, physicians, lifestyle therapists, and still, nothing works. Perhaps you already have a regimented pharmaceutical strategy for your hormonal imbalance and are looking to essential oils to supplement your treatment. Maybe you want to use essential oils exclusively in your journey to healing. Whatever your reason for reading this book, I am here to tell you that essential oils can help you and be a useful therapy for treating many different symptoms of hormonal imbalance. However, as with everything that can have a positive impact on the human body, essential oils can also have negative effects on the body. Therefore, it is important to consult a medical health professional before beginning any course of treatment involving essential oils. This book is merely a guide to essential oils and hormonal imbalance, and does not act as a self-diagnosing resource. While essential oils can be extremely helpful in treating the symptoms of hormonal imbalance, they do not necessarily treat the root cause of the imbalance. Using essential oils to mitigate the symptoms of anxiety, for example, a fast heart rate, intrusive thoughts, and feelings of impending doom, will not cure the cause of this anxiety. The causes of anxiety are varied and multifaceted and may be caused by anything from childhood trauma to stress at work. Before administering any essential oils, check with your doctor to see whether you are allergic to any of these substances. Perhaps, you have sensitive skin and must be aware of this before using essential oils. Once you have received the go-ahead, feel free to explore and use essential oils to your heart's content.

While essential oils probably won't help you heal your childhood trauma, they can provide a space of clarity and relief to promote healing. It is far more difficult to deal with your issues when you are overtired, overworked, and just trying to survive. Why would you want to improve your life if you can't even get up in the morning because you are exhausted and depressed? Essential oils can give you temporary relief. For example, peppermint oil can wake you up and revitalize you while lavender oil can put you to sleep. Your problems might not be solved, but you will be able to deal with them a little more constructively after a good night's rest. To best help you dive into the world of essential oils and hormone balance, this book is divided into three parts. Part 1 discusses the basics of essential oils and hormonal imbalance. In this section, you will find a comprehensive exploration of essential oils, their history, how they are made, and why they work. Did you know, even ancient Egyptians made use of essential oils? Civilizations from thousands of years B.C. have been crushing plants and using their oils for various treatments and tasks, so why shouldn't we do the same? Once you have a deeper understanding of essential oils and their place in ancient and modern society, you must use this information to learn about hormonal imbalance—how it can affect you at every stage of your life and how essential oils can help to rebalance and realign hormones. Hormone levels fluctuate at different stages of human life. For example, puberty refers to the increased release of hormones in the body during one's teenage years, while menopause refers to another hormonal shift at a later stage in life. It is important to recognize these fluctuations because you might just be entering a new stage in your physiological timeline. Sure, essential oils can still help you, but it is always nice to know why you might be experiencing these changes. Therefore, the chapter on hormonal imbalances will aim to clarify this process. In addition to exploring hormonal imbalance, the chapter will also delve into human anatomy to explain why we have hormones, what they do, where they come from, and why it is important to balance them.

Part 2 uses the knowledge gained in Part 1 and expands on it by exploring the different methods of using essential oils and how, when used effectively, these oils can help you mentally, spiritually, and physically. If you are wondering how you can improve your life to ensure that you are reaping the full benefits of essential oils, Part 2 provides a guide on how to use mindfulness, mediation, and creative visualization to promote the success of aromatherapy and essential oils. Part 2 also includes a comprehensive and detailed list of the most popular and useful essential oils. This chapter will highlight the ingredients, benefits, uses, best practices, and tips and tricks for each essential oil. Whenever you have a problem, you can just scroll through the guide and find the right oil for you. For example, if you feel restless and are struggling to sleep, you can check out Chapter 6, read through the list of essential oils and find that lavender oil is the right oil for the occasion. It is also useful to have an encyclopaedic understanding of essential oils because it will allow you to understand how each oil can help to treat symptoms in its own unique way.

Once you know about the oils and how to use them, it is time to move on to Part 3. Here, you will learn about different hormonal imbalances and which essential oils should be used to treat symptoms. Whether you are experiencing physiological, mental, or other symptoms caused by hormonal imbalance, these chapters will describe the symptoms, prescribe the most suitable essential oil for treatment, and offer advice on how to best use or apply the oil for maximum effectiveness. Once you have been transformed into an essential oil guru, Chapter 11 contains a 14-day detoxifying essential oil guide to show you how you can use essential oils in your everyday life and get your mind, body, and soul ready for essential oil therapy. Essential oils can be used in self-care practices, but on a more practical level, some essential oils are also antifungal and antiseptic which means that they can be used in first aid treatment and in cleaning practices.

Essential oils can be life-changing if you give them the opportunity and space to work. However, they are also not a magical cure that will make all of your problems go away. To get the best results one must use essential oils to their full potential. Imagine injuring your knee and getting surgery to fix it. After a few weeks, it feels good, but you fail to go to any of the post-operative physiotherapy appointments. The knee, while it feels stable, probably won't heal fully. Having surgery is not a miracle cure (in many cases it is, but that is not without the necessary pre- and post-operative therapies). Similarly, essential oil therapy is not a miracle cure. Living an unhealthy lifestyle and expecting essential oils to make everything right is a little on the unrealistic side. But fear not because, in this book, I will give you all of the tools and strategies necessary for living a holistic and healthy life with the help of essential oils. But first, what are essential oils?

Part 1:

The Basics of Essential Oils and Hormonal Imbalance

Chapter 1

What Are Essential Oils?

Essential oils are extracts from plants. They are often referred to as the *essence* of a plant. Plants are pressed, steamed, or put through various other processes to extract the unique compounds that make them distinctive. For example, lavender has a very specific scent and chemical compound that has calming properties. The essence of lavender is extracted as a concentrated form of the plant's distinctive qualities. Think of it like an artichoke. To get to the juicy, flavorful heart of the artichoke you have to peel off many leaves and layers. Similarly, when you want to get to the essence of a plant, you have to remove the excess water, leaves, and flowers until you have a pure compound, also known as an essential oil.

Throughout your life as a human, you will inevitably ask yourself the question *who am I?* It is a question that plagues humanity at every corner as people try to decipher who it is they are at their very core. While that question may feel unreachable and nebulous, imagine if you could carry around a small vial of what it means to be you. Gone would be the days of doubting and second-guessing yourself. You would know who and why you are, and would be able to walk through life confidently and without hesitation.

Essential oils are exactly that. They are the quintessence of plants.

Essential oils are extracted from plants through their flowers, seeds, stems, leaves, fruits, and branches. Depending on the plant, the extraction method will be different. For example, oranges store their essential oils in the peel, while lavender stores its essential oils in its flowers and leaves. Not all plants produce essential oils and that is why the practice of using essential oils is so specialized. For many years, people have tried and tested extracts of various plants to decipher which plants are best suited for certain purposes. This is what makes essential oils so fascinating. They are not extracted and used at random. They have been explored for thousands of years to be known and used as the oils that we know and love today. Yes, there are skeptics and no, essential oils won't cure all of your trauma and financial issues. But the reason they are still around today is that they work and can help you. And, if thousands of years of practice and testing is not testament enough to their effectiveness, plants actually use their own essential oils. They use these naturally occurring oils to help with "infection control, humidity control, hormonal effects, wound healing, and attracting or repelling insects, birds, and animals" (Halcon, n.d.). If nature can do that for itself, imagine what it can do for you.

Aromatherapy is a word often used to describe the effects that scents may have on the body. The human brain uses smell to recall memories and emotions. It's like when you walk past a bakery and remember the smell of the cake your mom baked every Sunday morning. Immediately, just by encountering a slightly doughy and sweet scent, you are transported back in time. Scents are powerful and they have a significant impact on how humans interact with the world. Therefore, aromatherapy is the practice of using aromatics (like essential oils) to holistically improve mental, spiritual, and physical wellbeing.

Today, human beings like to think of themselves as more evolved than past generations. The fact of the matter is that, while we have made major technological advancements, we can still benefit greatly from nature and everything it has to offer. Just because it comes from nature does not mean that we need to brush it off as ineffective quackery. Similar to how eating vegetables and having a balanced diet will improve your health and provide your body with the nutrients it needs to survive; essential oils can do the same. Just because they don't have robotic arms or a modern aesthetic does not mean we should turn our backs on natural resources.

A Brief History of Essential Oils

As long as plants and humans coexist, essential oils will most likely be used. Similar to how we use nature to nourish our bodies, essential oils nourish our minds, bodies, and souls. Unsurprisingly, cultures throughout history have used essential oils for that very purpose. One of the oldest *known* uses of essential oils is in ancient Egypt. The ancient Egyptians used essential oils for a plethora of different purposes but one of the most interesting uses was to incorporate them in the embalming process. While they included essential oils in the embalming process to mask the odor of decomposition, they also used myrrh to stop bacteria and fungus from growing. In addition to this, the ancient Egyptians used essential oils for hygiene purposes, as perfume, in religion, cosmetics, and medicinally. The anti-microbial properties of essential oils were used to fight off pathogens and certain insects in ancient Egypt, but they also used these oils to soften their skin. The first evidence of the use of essential oils is believed to be dated as far back as 10,000 B.C.; however, more definitive evidence details the presence of essential oils closer to 5000 B.C.

After the ancient Egyptians, the use of essential oils is present in Chinese and Indian culture in around 3000-2000 B.C. Although, there is evidence showing the Chinese and ancient Egyptians using essential oils at roughly the same time. The Ebers Papyrus and the Nei Ching are two of the oldest known medical journals that still exist today. The former was discovered in ancient Egypt and includes the use of essential oils in its doctrine. It also includes information about pregnancy and determining the sex of a child before birth. It is an incredibly advanced journal for its time. The Nei Ching dictates that balance and returning to balance are the key factors to health. It states that this can be done using *Qi* (life force), *Yin* (negative forces), and *Yang* (positive forces), as well as *Wuxing*, also known as the five phases which include, fire, water, wood, metal, and earth (Hafner, n.d.). These doctrines, being so interlinked with nature, involved the exploration of essential oils and other healing techniques, such as acupuncture. In addition to this, Shen Nung, also known as the father of Chinese medicine, wrote a book detailing the effects and uses of 300 different plants and herbs. In his exploration of these plants and herbs, he died from poisoning. His dedication to essential oils and plants is why we can use these oils safely and securely today.

Similarly, in India, one of the oldest religions in the world makes use of essential oils. The Ayurvedic religion promotes balance in aspects of diet, lifestyle, and consciousness. One of the aspects of Ayurveda is the function of nature, which is made up of three elements, mainly *Kapha*, *Pitta*, and *Vata*. These elements consist of fire, air, water, and space. When one of these functions is off-balance, specific essential oils are used to return to equilibrium. For example, *Vata* deals with space and air elements and can bring about dryness and coldness. Therefore, to be treated, one can use essential oils like sage, cinnamon, and cloves to counteract the effects of the imbalance. In this sense, the religious uses of essential oils also play a very practical and medicinal role in healing and worship. What can be learnt from the use of essential oils by the Chinese and the Indians is the desire to bring balance and return to equilibrium.

Roughly 1500 years later, in 400 B.C., Hippocrates started to research the use of essential oils in Ancient Greece. Known as the father of medicine, Hippocrates changed the way we view medicine. Even today, every doctor has to swear by the Hippocratic oath before they are qualified to practice medicine. Hippocrates believed in the concept of holism. Essentially, holism encourages the entire being to return to equilibrium. By viewing the human body as an entire organism which is constantly acting and reacting to different changes and stimuli, one can treat the body as a whole and not just as part of an organism. Hippocrates believed that daily baths and massages with essential oils were the keys to living a healthy lifestyle. Apart from this, his belief in the healing properties of nature allowed him to rid Greece of a plague. He used essential oils to fumigate the city center because of their antibacterial properties (International Federation of Aromatherapists, n.d.). The practice of using essential oils eventually reached the Romans where they continued to add to the already well-researched index of herbs and plants. The Romans passed their knowledge down to the British Isles who used essential oils as perfumes.

There is evidence of the use of essential oils in early Christianity and Islam. The old and new testaments refer to myrrh and an anointing oil which was made from several essential oils, including cinnamon. The presence of these oils in Christianity defined their presence in Western society. However, during the time of the bubonic plague, essential oils were used to mask the smell of decay. They were also used for their antifungal and antibacterial properties. As time went on, essential oils were consistently used as perfumes. These oils gained popularity and, by the 17th century, they were so widely used that their long history of medical healing became farcical and distrusted. Because they were so popular and widely available, people found ways to cheat the system to make extra money. They would add filler ingredients to the oils and sell them under false pretenses, making the whole business generally unreliable.

However, this was instigated by the Catholic Church as they began to threaten and demonize midwives for their use of essential oils and natural products to aid in menstruation, menopause, childbirth, birth control, and abortion practices. The Catholic Church villainized these practices and labeled them as witchcraft. This set medicine back a few years as it neglected the medical treatment of female bodies and also transformed medical practice into a space exclusively reserved for the male members of the church. After this, natural medicinal practices and essential oils were relegated to perfumes and cosmetics. That is until scientists began synthetically reproducing the compounds of essential oils. As chemistry and modern pharmaceuticals started developing, scientists began pulling apart the chemical compounds of essential oils to produce them in labs. In the late 19th century, scientists found that people working with and processing flowers were not susceptible to respiratory diseases. They also found that essential oils could fight off microorganisms from yellow fever to glandular fever. By understanding the capabilities and advantages of essential oils, scientists used these qualities to replicate the chemical structures and use these compounds in modern medicine.

Natural essential oils, once again, gained traction, thanks to Rene Maurice Gattefosse, the inventor of aromatherapy and a chemist who discovered the effectiveness of lavender oil after he suffered a serious burn on his hand. He found that his hand healed exceptionally quickly which led him to embark on further research into essential oils and their healing properties. Essential oils today are seen as an effective supplementary treatment in medicine and they have made their mark on the medical community. You can find these oils in almost every pharmacy and chemist in the world. Thanks to years of research, trials, and testing, essential oils, as we know them today, are available and at your disposal.

How Are Essential Oils Made?

There are several different methods used to extract essential oils from plants. Some of these methods are more effective than others. Some are tailored to specific plants to optimize extraction. Understanding how essential oils are extracted will allow you to better decide which processes provide the purest form of oil while giving you the confidence to know and understand where your essential oils come from. Some of these methods include:

Steam Distillation

This is one of the most popular methods of extraction because it does not require any additional ingredients or reactors to extract the desired material. The end result is, therefore, relatively pure. Steam distillation works by placing the plant material (i.e., the seeds, leaves, flowers, etc.) into a vessel and passing vaporized water through them. The steam causes the plant material to release some of its oils and carries these oils up and over to another vessel. In the second vessel, the hot air escapes from an opening while cold water is used to cool the steam and trap the condensation. Essential oils are highly volatile compounds which means that they can evaporate. This is why the process of steam distillation works so well. Once the essential oils and water have condensed, the liquid moves to a separator wherein the water is removed and the essential oils are left in pure form. This process of extraction produces an organic product which means the essential oils are 100% pure and solvent-free. It allows the oil to be used in the most effective and successful way. While this method is widely used, not all essential oils can be extracted in this manner and, therefore, require different methods for successful extraction.

Cold Press

This method is designed to extract oils from fruits, specifically oranges and lemons, as their essential oils are found in the skin and rind of the fruit. To extract these oils, the fruit is placed in a machine that pierces the skin on the fruit to release the essential oils. After the skin is pierced, the whole fruit is pressed to release any excess oils and juices. The pulp is then removed from the liquid and the oil is separated from the juice in a separator. The oil is then extracted and ready to be bottled. While the name of this method is deceiving, the term actually refers to the fact that the temperatures to which the plant material is exposed should not exceed 80 degrees Fahrenheit. This contrasts with the steam distillation method, which requires heat to extract the necessary oils. However, similar to the steam distillation method, cold pressing also means that the essential oil is in its purest and most organic form because it is solvent-free and has not undergone any additional chemical processes. The absence of heat also means that the essential oil may retain more of its structure and value. Similar to how vegetables lose some of their nutrients in the cooking process, plants may lose some of their oils in the heating process.

Maceration

This process involves using a carrier oil to extract essential oils from a plant. This works better than steam distillation because the carrier oil allows heavier particles to be included in the essential oil. Water cannot extract or carry these heavier particles because it is not dense enough. Maceration is slightly more complex than steam distillation or cold press extraction. It involves using plants in their driest form because water can cause the extract to become rancid. Once the plant material is dried, it is finely cut. This process helps to break down the cell walls of the plant and allows for maximum extraction. Once the plant material is dried and cut, it is placed in an airtight vessel with a solvent. This solvent can be used to dissolve some of the plant material so it can become part of the essential oil. While this process does make use of a solvent and is not 100% pure or organic, it allows for more of the plant material to be incorporated into the extract. This solvent and plant mixture can sit for several days. The mixture should be stirred every day. Then, the extract is removed and the rest of the plant solids are pressed to ensure all of the oil has been extracted. After this, the liquid is filtered and ready for use.

Carbon Dioxide Extraction

Carbon dioxide extraction is the most interesting and recent method of essential oil extraction that has been developed. While it has not been extensively researched and we cannot know if it has harmful side effects, we can understand that carbon dioxide is an element which is required by most living creatures. After all, humans breathe out carbon dioxide and plants require it to survive and photosynthesize. The use of carbon dioxide also means that the extraction process is mostly environmentally friendly, and produces organic and pure essential oil.

The extraction process involves pressurizing carbon dioxide so that it becomes *supercritical*, which means that it is converted into liquid form. The pressurized liquid form of carbon dioxide is mixed with the plant material and causes the essential oil to dissolve into the carbon dioxide. From here, the liquid is depressurized and the carbon dioxide returns to its gaseous state, evaporating from the oil and leaving a pure essential oil as the final product. The reason this process is so revolutionary is that it does not alter the natural state of the plant material or essential oil. Instead, it acts as a harmless solvent which leads to an organic essential oil. In addition to carbon dioxide acting as a natural solvent, the process does not employ heat as liberally as steam distillation does. By heating the plant material at a high temperature, a lot of the oil constituents can be lost which results in a less concentrated essential oil.

Carbon dioxide extraction, while not on the same level as the cold press method, does not exceed temperatures of 100 degrees Fahrenheit and, therefore, does not alter the plant materials or the extracted oils. This also means that the final product is often thicker and more concentrated than with any other method of extraction.

Enfleurage

This is one of the oldest methods of essential oil extraction. While it is not commonly used today, it can be used to make essential oils at home. Enfleurage involves using an odorless fat which is solid at room temperature. Lard and other animal fat products are often used. The fat is laid out and the plant material is pressed into the animal fat. The process is repeated every few days and the old plant material is removed. Once the desired saturation is reached, alcohol is added to separate the animal fat from the plant oil and the essential oil is extracted. Often, the leftover animal fat is used to make soap, which means this method serves a dual purpose. In the same way that you might add essential oils to creams or carrier oils, this soap can also be utilized as a method for hormone balance.

Water Distillation

This method is very similar to the steam distillation method except it submerges delicate plant material into water to protect it from overheating. This method works well when delicate leaves and flowers are involved. Basically, the plant material is submerged in water and the plant oils are released into the water. Think of it like making tea. When you put a teabag into hot water and leave it there for a few minutes, the water takes on the flavor of the tea leaves and also changes color. In a similar way, submerging the plant material into hot (but not too hot) water will allow the necessary oils and essences to be extracted. From here, the steam and water distillation processes are relatively similar. The water gets heated up to around 140 degrees Fahrenheit and the steam picks up and moves the oils to another vessel where they are cooled and condensation occurs. The mixture moves into a separator where the oil and water are separated and the essential oil is extracted.

Solvent Distillation

Solvent distillation, while effective, produces the least concentrated essential oil. However, it is very useful for plants that do not yield a large amount of essential oils. Solvent distillation works by mixing the plant material with alcohol or a similar type of solvent. This mixture extracts wax and oil from the plant material. The wax and oil mixture is heated to remove the alcohol. Once the alcohol is removed, the oil is evaporated and passes through a vessel containing cold water to promote condensation. The condensate is filtered and the essential oil is extracted. While this method has its upsides, it does produce an extract that is not organic and does contain solvents. In this way, some of the other methods result in a better, more concentrated, and purer essential oil, but solvent distillation is perfect for perfumes due to the alcohol content.

While it is important to understand how essential oils are extracted, it is also important to understand how this process can go wrong. To reap the full benefits of essential oils, they have to be 100% pure. Here are some factors that may influence the quality of essential oils during production:

Contamination

Contamination is a huge issue in the extraction of essential oils. Contamination can occur at any point in the extraction process. Whether it is due to human error, improper sanitation, or inferior heating processes contamination is a risk. For example, with maceration extraction, if there is too much water present in the plant material, then the essential oil will become rancid. If people handle the essential oils without the proper protective gear and sterilized equipment then bacteria can alter the profile of the essential oil. If the machinery and equipment are not thoroughly cleaned, then the oil can be contaminated with other or older essential oils. Contamination can also occur during harvest. If the plant material has been sprayed with pesticides or growth hormones, then the end result will be a synthetic and contaminated essential oil that may affect you negatively. This is why using a trustworthy brand can make all the difference to your essential oil experience. Read reviews, study the processes, and decide which essential oil provider is the safest, cleanest, and purest before rushing into any decisions.

Adulteration

This is when something is added that reduces the purity of the oil. If an oil is adulterated, it means that it is not entirely made up of the essential oil but contains other ingredients. Often companies will add alcohol or carrier oils to increase the amount of essential oil; however, this reduces the purity and, therefore, results in an inferior product. As I said before, figuring out which brand to use can help to prevent this. Reduced purity means that you won't be able to reap the full benefits of the essential oil and your experience may be lackluster. To avoid this, make sure the products are 100% organic and approved by a professional. This will ensure that you are getting the product you paid for.

Harvested at the Right Time

This factor includes a few other variables. Not only must the plant material be harvested at the correct time, but depending on whether or not the season's weather was opportune, this will inevitably alter the quality and profile of the essential oil. For example, if plant material is harvested too early, it might not be mature enough to provide the optimal concentration for the essential oil. Similarly, if the plant is harvested too late, the number of nutrients it contains may be fewer than necessary and the oil may not be as rich. Things like soil and nitrogen levels also influence the quality of the essential oil. Have you ever wondered why wines are different every year? Each brand has a specific Chardonnay or Merlot for every year. This is because the season changes, the soil is different, the crops are new, and there are so many variables when it comes to nature and weather. Each production cycle could be different. Try to keep track of where the plant material was harvested, how the oil was extracted, and how these variables can affect essential oil products. Also, factors like storage times can be very influential regarding the quality of an essential oil. If the oil has gone through the maceration process of extraction, then it will only be usable for six to twelve months. If the product is being stored in a factory for six months then you only have another six months to use it. There are many variables but once you find a brand that you trust, your essential oil journey will bring you nothing but joy and balance.

Does It Work?

While there has been a lot of historical evidence pertaining to the success and efficacy of essential oils, there is yet to be detailed scientific evidence regarding the efficacy of these plant extracts. It is true; humans have relied on and utilized plants for thousands of years and if they were not in some way effective, their popularity would have dwindled. However, this evidence is circumstantial and does not depict the true scientific properties or success of essential oils. One might wonder why lavender oils have relaxing properties or why sage oil can help with inflammation. It's kind of like when you hear a grammatically incorrect sentence. You can identify the error and correct it, but you don't really know why it is incorrect. Similarly, one can say that certain essential oils help with certain ailments but there is little scientific research telling us why. However, the field of essential oil research is not totally barren. Here are a few studies that have proven the efficacy of essential oils:

Antifungal and Antibacterial Efficacy

There have been several scientific studies conducted with regards to the antifungal and antibacterial properties of essential oils. One of the first studies, conducted in 1887, tested the effects of essential oils against tuberculosis and other respiratory diseases. It was confirmed that essential oils played a hand in curing glandular fever and yellow fever. Using these results, scientists from the Technical University of Denmark conducted an experiment testing the antifungal properties of certain oils. They soaked rye bread in essential oils and determined the level of spoilage. They found that clove, thyme, and cinnamon were the best inhibitors of fungal growth while orange, sage, and rosemary did not exhibit the same efficacy in terms of inhibiting fungal growth (Suhr, 2003). These studies also resulted in findings that showed when essential oils were most effective. Thyme, clove, and cinnamon were found to be most effective when applied directly to the rye bread, while mustard and lemongrass were most effective when applied with a carrier oil. These findings, while not far-reaching in terms of the essential oils explored, confirm that some essential oils do have antifungal and antibacterial properties.

Dementia

A study was conducted involving 72 patients who suffered from severe dementia. Seventy-one of the candidates completed the trial. The tests were done using lemon balm. There was a 35% improvement in the symptoms of dementia and an overall increase in the quality of life (Ballard, 2002). While this study does not confirm that lemon balm cures dementia, it did lead to an overall improvement in the symptoms experienced and generally helped people suffering from dementia.

Acne

Tests were conducted to determine the efficacy of tea tree oil in curing acne. The test included 60 participants, half of which used tea tree oil and the other half of which used a placebo oil. It was found that tea tree oil was five times more effective than the placebo gel and is, therefore, considered an effective and safe cure for acne (Enshaieh, 2007).

Alopecia

Scientists successfully treated people who had been diagnosed with alopecia. Eighty-six participants were tested for seven months. Forty-three participants had to rub essential oils (such as thyme, cedarwood, lavender, and rosemary) added to a carrier oil into their scalp daily. The remaining 41 participants used carrier oil. The results showed a noticeable difference in the group using essential oils. The results were evaluated by two independent dermatologists who used photographs to highlight the before-and-after effects of the treatment. They concluded that essential oils and aromatherapy are useful treatments for alopecia (Hay, 1998).

Antibacterial and Anti-Inflammatory

One study, which used mice to test the anti-inflammatory properties of citrus oil found that, when combined with Dead Sea salt and used at the right concentration, citrus oil was successful in inhibiting bacterial growth and also reduced inflammation in the mice (Mizrahi, 2006).

Food Poisoning

One study found that essential oils, like bergamot, could stop the spread of bacteria that causes food poisoning. They found that it successfully inhibited the growth of listeria, E. coli, and staphylococcus bacteria (Fisher, 2006).

Essential oils have many different purposes and properties and the ones mentioned above are only the oils that have been scientifically tested. The reason that structured testing for essential oils has been under-researched is that the oils are not consistent. As mentioned earlier, just as wine is different every year due to ever-changing variables, so are the plants that produce essential oils. In this way, testing can be unreliable. However, while the effects of essential oils have not been entirely tested or proven, there is enough research and history to confirm that essential oils can be used for holistic healing.

Chapter 2

What Is Hormonal Imbalance?

To determine what hormonal imbalances are and what they look like, it is crucial to have a basic understanding of the human body and the glands and hormones that help it to function. Yes, this chapter may use some words you have never heard before; however, this is not your standard biology lesson. Instead of walking away confused and befuddled, you will be able to confidently strut to the next chapter with a comprehensive understanding of how the human body works and how essential oils can help with hormonal imbalances. So, let's start with the basics:

What is a Gland?

The body has two glandular systems—the endocrine system and the exocrine system. The endocrine system consists of ductless glands that release hormones into the bloodstream. The exocrine system is made up of glands that release substances through a duct. An example of an exocrine gland is the sweat gland. The substances released by the exocrine system are not hormones and, therefore, are not considered to be part of the endocrine system. By definition, "A gland is an organ in the body which produces and releases substances that perform a specific function in the body" (Your Hormones, n.d.). The substances released by the endocrine system are known as hormones.

What is a Hormone?

A hormone is a chemical that is produced by specific parts of the body within the endocrine system. These chemicals help the body to function as it needs to so that it can grow and survive. Essentially, hormones act as a means of communication between the different parts of the body. For example, when the growth hormone is released, it sends signals to other parts of the body and tells them to grow. However, sometimes it is not as simple as that. For the growth hormone to be activated, a different gland has to release a growth hormone-releasing hormone. Suddenly, there is a very complex and well-orchestrated system of communication happening inside of your body without you being aware of what is happening. There are many different hormones with many different functions. Understanding how their balance or subsequent imbalance can affect you and your body will help you on the journey to healing.

So, what does it mean when a hormone is imbalanced? An imbalance occurs when there is too much or too little of something. As I said, your hormones are perfectly orchestrated chemicals which are released at specific times. If the timing or structure of these chemicals are skewed to one side, it can result in a vast array of physiological, physical, and mental symptoms and conditions. To understand hormonal imbalance, you must be aware of the different hormones and their functions within the body.

Pineal Gland

The pineal gland is located at the center of the brain between the two hemispheres. It secretes melatonin and serotonin and can be found in most vertebrates. If the pineal gland is damaged or inhibited, this can lead to hormonal imbalance which often results in insomnia.

- Melatonin

This hormone deals with sleep and the body's circadian cycle. It is often referred to as the *sleep hormone*. It uses the brain's interpretation of time to follow a day/night pattern and also functions seasonally, releasing more melatonin during winter months as the nights become longer. Melatonin works with light and dark. The brain interprets light through the eyes and responds accordingly. If the eyes are exposed to light, the pineal gland will not release melatonin. If the eyes are not exposed to light, the pineal gland will release melatonin to encourage sleep. This is why you may find that you fall asleep quicker if you stop using a phone or laptop 30 minutes before bed. The light from the screens filters in through the eyes which send signals to the pineal gland. The pineal gland does not release enough melatonin because it interprets the light as daylight. During sleep, the pineal gland releases ten times more melatonin than during the day. This helps to maintain sleep. Although melatonin is not essential for sleep, it does aid in the process. If there is too much melatonin in your system, you can feel tired and drowsy. If there is too little, you might experience insomnia or haphazard sleeping schedules.

- Serotonin

Serotonin, also known as the *happiness hormone* is secreted by the pineal gland. While most people know serotonin for its mood-improving qualities, it also helps with sleep, nausea, and bowel movements. Serotonin regulates mood and is released when exercising or doing things you enjoy. If one has too little serotonin, this can result in depression, anxiety, and insomnia. If one has too much serotonin, this may lead to feelings of restlessness and high blood pressure. It can also decrease bone density and cause osteoporosis. For these reasons, it is crucial to keep your hormones balanced as the imbalance could lead to serious health problems.

Pituitary Gland

This is one of the most important glands in the human body. It controls the functions of all the other glands in the endocrine system. It also controls growth and development. It is located under the brain, behind the nose, at the base of the skull. Part of the pituitary gland is attached to the hypothalamus which is a part of the brain that is also considered a gland. Because the pituitary gland controls the functions of many other glands and hormones, it is difficult to pinpoint all of the things that can go wrong when these hormones are imbalanced. However, some of the most common symptoms and conditions occurring due to imbalance include acromegaly (a condition caused by an excess of the growth hormone that leads to increased bone size) and diabetes.

- Adrenocorticotropic hormone

This hormone is crucial to the function of the adrenal gland as it activates the release of cortisol which is used to activate the body's stress response. If there is too much of this hormone in the body it can lead to tumor growth. Having too little of the hormone can lead to a loss of appetite, nausea, and weakness.

- Follicle-stimulating hormone

This hormone stimulates the growth of follicles in the ovaries so that eggs can attach to the uterine lining. It also stimulates the growth of cells that promote sperm production in the testes. If there is too little of this hormone in the body, it can lead to an incomplete puberty and even infertility. If there is too much of the follicle-stimulating hormone, it can also lead to infertility and a lowered sex drive.

- Growth hormone

This hormone contributes to growth and development throughout a person's life. It promotes growth in children and during puberty but works to maintain normal body structure in adults. If there is too much of this hormone in the body, it can lead to conditions like gigantism. Too little of the hormone can result in a weakened body structure, a weak heart, and increased fat.

- Prolactin

Prolactin deals with the production of breast milk during pregnancy and after childbirth. If there is too much prolactin in the body, it could result in the excess production of milk and irregular menstrual periods. If there is too little of the hormone, it can lead to insufficient milk production after childbirth.

- Thyroid-stimulating hormone

The thyroid-stimulating hormone regulates the hormones produced by the thyroid. If there is too much of this hormone, it can be indicative of an overactive thyroid while having too little can suggest an underactive thyroid.

- Luteinising hormone

This hormone is responsible for the reproductive functions of the body. For men, it stimulates the production of testosterone which, in turn, produces sperm. For women, it is present throughout the menstrual cycle. It stimulates and releases follicles to increase the chances of pregnancy. If there is too much or too little of this hormone, it can result in infertility.

- Melanocyte-stimulating hormone

This hormone controls pigmentation, provides protection from the sun, and controls appetite. If there is too much in your body, this can lead to hyperpigmentation. If there is too little, it can lead to a lack of pigmentation and inadequate protection against UV rays.

Thyroid Gland

The thyroid gland controls the metabolic functions of the body. To do this, it controls the digestive muscles, heart, and brain development to provide constant and healthy metabolic function throughout the body. Iodine is a big contributor to thyroid health, therefore, controlling your diet allows you to take care of your thyroid and prevent some of the symptoms of imbalance. Having an overactive thyroid (known as hyperthyroidism) can lead to weight loss, nervousness, a fast heart rate, and sleep problems. In contrast, having an underactive thyroid (referred to as hypothyroidism) can lead to weight gain, drowsiness, slow heart rate, and forgetfulness.

- Triiodothyronine

Triiodothyronine is one of the two hormones produced by the thyroid gland. It contributes to the functioning of the metabolism, as well as bone and brain development and function. This hormone, also known as T3, makes up 20% of the hormones released by the thyroid gland. Having too much or too little of this hormone results in the previously mentioned conditions of hyperthyroidism and hypothyroidism.

- Thyroxine

This hormone (also known as T4) makes up 80% of the hormones released by the thyroid gland; however, when it reaches the liver and kidneys, it is transformed into T3. This hormone functions in the same way as triiodothyronine except it is considered to be the inactive version.

Parathyroid Gland

This gland controls the levels of calcium in the body. It is located behind the thyroid gland and works closely with the kidneys to regulate calcium levels. It also ensures that bone strength is built up and maintained.

- Parathormone

The parathormone is the only hormone produced by the parathyroid gland. It is released when the body experiences a shortage of calcium. It works to increase calcium absorption in the intestines and also reduces the amount of calcium excreted in urine. Too much parathormone can lead to an excess of calcium. This can result in kidney disease and a vitamin D deficiency. Too little of the parathyroid gland leads to depression, anxiety, tiredness, and brain fog.

Adrenal Gland

These glands are located at the top of each kidney and serve as a messenger to other hormones and glands to make sure everything is functioning properly. The adrenal glands are structured into two layers—the outer layer, known as the adrenal cortex, and the inner layer, known as the adrenal medulla. The cortex produces cortisol, aldosterone, and adrenal androgens, and the medulla produces catecholamines.

- Cortisol

Also known as the *stress hormone*, plays a significant role in fighting off illnesses and inflammation. It also helps to regulate the metabolism. Too much cortisol can result in weight gain, high blood pressure, osteoporosis, and weakened muscles. If there is too little cortisol in the body, one can experience weight loss, fatigue, and weakened muscles.

- Aldosterone

This is a very important hormone as it controls and regulates the salt and water levels of the body. If there is too little aldosterone, then one might experience low blood pressure and dehydration. If there is too much, it can cause the body to retain too much salt, ultimately leading to high blood pressure.

- Adrenal androgens

Dehydroepiandrosterone and testosterone are adrenal androgens and they are mainly male sex hormones. Too much of these hormones can lead to increased muscle mass and hair growth, baldness, and acne in both males and females. Having too little of these hormones can result in inadequate development and infertility.

- Catecholamines

These include adrenaline and dopamine and work in conjunction with cortisol to simulate a stress response. Too much of these hormones can lead to increased sweating, heart palpitations, and high blood pressure. Too little of these can reduce the effectiveness of a stress response.

Hypothalamus

The hypothalamus is a part of the brain which regulates the body and maintains homeostasis. This means that it ensures the body is kept stable at all times. In this way, it makes sense that it controls temperature, sex drive, sleep, hunger, thirst, and energy. So, if you feel hungry or thirsty, the hypothalamus responds by sending signals to the brain and body telling you to eat so that the body can return to homeostasis. Additionally, the hypothalamus deals with memory and stress responses.

- Somatostatin

This hormone stops the production of certain hormones in the body like the pancreatic hormones and growth hormones. If there is too much somatostatin, it can lead to diabetes and gallstones. If there is too little, it can lead to an overproduction of the growth hormone.

- Oxytocin

Oxytocin is released during childbirth and lactation and also plays an important role in social behavior. If there is too much oxytocin in the body, it can lead to emotional sensitivity and prostate enlargement. Having too little can lead to depression and inhibit the ejection of milk during breastfeeding.

- Thyrotropin-releasing hormone

This hormone regulates thyroid activity. There have been no known cases of someone having too much of this hormone; however, too little can lead to an underactive thyroid.

- Growth hormone-releasing hormone

This hormone stimulates the pituitary gland to release the growth hormone into the body. Too much of the growth hormone-releasing hormone can lead to ectopic tumors, gigantism, and diabetes. Having too little can lead to growth deficiency and inadequate development.

Ovaries

The ovaries control female reproduction and menstruation. They are located on either side of the uterus and are used to store and release eggs.

- Estrogen

Estrogen aids in development throughout puberty and regulates the menstrual cycle. It also helps with childbearing and regulates cholesterol. If there is too little estrogen in the body, it can lead to dryness, irregular periods, and increased urinary tract infections. Too much estrogen can lead to weight gain, irregular periods, and may even cause thyroid dysfunction.

- Progesterone

This is one of the two hormones released by the ovaries. Progesterone regulates pregnancy and menstrual cycles as it prepares the body for pregnancy. Often, people who have high levels of progesterone in their bodies suffer from breast cancer. A lack of progesterone can lead to polycystic ovary syndrome and an inability to carry a pregnancy to term.

Pancreas

The pancreas aids in food digestion and regulates glucose levels in the blood.

- Insulin

Insulin is released by the pancreas to regulate glucose levels in the blood. If there is too much or too little insulin, it can lead to diabetes.

- Glucagon

Glucagon also regulates glucose levels in the body and makes sure the glucose levels remain stable by engaging the liver in glucose production.

- Gastrin

Gastrin produces gastric acid to aid in food digestion. Too much gastrin in the body can lead to ulcers or diarrhea due to the excess of gastric acid. If there is too little gastrin in the body, one might experience an increased risk of infection as the lack of acid can no longer kill off harmful bacteria.

Testes

The testes are the male reproductive glands which produce sperm and testosterone.

- Testosterone

Testosterone plays a part in male reproduction as well as muscle development. If there is too much testosterone, it can lead to acne, baldness, and infertility. If there is too little testosterone in the body, one might experience infertility and a decreased sex drive.

Thymus

The thymus gland stops working after puberty; however, it has long-lasting effects on the body even after it has ceased production. It works to increase autoimmunity and fight off diseases.

- Thymosin

Thymosin stimulates the production of T cells which are essential in fighting off diseases. Since production stops after puberty, the rate of imbalance is low.

Hormonal Imbalance: A Timeline

Hormones can be confusing and frustrating but they are also incredibly helpful and, well, our survival as human beings depends on them. Once you understand what they are, why they are, what they do, and how they change throughout your life, it can be easier to regulate, maintain, and even appreciate them for everything they do. Understanding your body at all of its different stages can help you to figure out what kind of imbalances you may be experiencing and why. For this reason, I have created a hormonal timeline of what to expect and what to watch out for as you go through life.

Pre-Puberty

During this time, everything is pretty normal. Your hormones are stable, the growth hormone is doing its job, the thymus is producing some T cells and your body has the whole survival thing under control. However, at this stage of development, the ovaries and testes are not producing hormones yet.

Puberty

This starts between the ages of 8–13 for girls and 9–14 for boys. At this time, the hypothalamus produces gonadotropin, a hormone that stimulates the production and release of estrogen and testosterone. The luteinizing and follicle-stimulating hormones are also released at this stage. This causes changes like the development of breasts and other sex organs, the growth of pubic hair, the deepening of the voice, and increased growth. Puberty can be a tumultuous time for most teenagers as it comes with a few embarrassing symptoms. The hormonal imbalance catalyzed by puberty can also cause acne, mood swings, and fatigue.

Post-Puberty

After the influx of hormones, the body takes a few years to acclimate and reach a stable and regular level of functioning. By now, hormone levels have stabilized, periods are regular, growth has stopped, and reproductive organs are fully developed. Remember, it is at this stage that the thymus stops producing T cells; however, this should have little to no effect on hormonal imbalance. For females during menstruation, the levels of estrogen and progesterone fluctuate to increase the chances of pregnancy.

Perimenopause

Perimenopause occurs in women prior to the age of 50. It is a gradual built up to full-blown menopause. Perimenopause starts between the ages of 40 and 50. At this stage, menstruation becomes more irregular and the production of progesterone and estrogen decreases, leading to a lowered sex drive, vaginal dryness, and night sweats.

Menopause

Menopause usually occurs in women at around the age of 50 and refers to the hormonal changes happening in the body. Menstruation stops at this stage. Usually, the production of estrogen and progesterone decreases because childbearing becomes less frequent as one ages. This change in hormone levels can lead to hot flashes, insomnia, a decreased sex drive, and depression.

Andropause

This is similar to menopause but is not an exact equivalent. For starters, not all men experience andropause. But the ones that do may notice a decreased sex drive, decreased muscle mass, and even erectile dysfunction. It is in these stages of life, while natural and expected, that one must try to combat and treat the symptoms of hormonal imbalance.

Pregnancy

Similarly to puberty, gonadotropin is also released during pregnancy to ensure the growth of the fetus. Progesterone and estrogen production increase to ensure the success of the pregnancy. Symptoms of hormonal imbalance during pregnancy can include mood swings, swelling, and cravings. However, these symptoms are considered normal during this stage.

How Essential Oils Can Help

As you have learnt by now, the balance of hormones is crucial to the functioning of the human body. If these hormones are even a little off-balance, the body notices and reacts to the changes. While there are supplements and medications available, the symptoms of hormonal imbalance can still be harsh and debilitating. This is why using an alternative method of treatment, like essential oils and aromatherapy, can be extremely useful to any situation involving hormonal imbalance.

In the previous chapter, the effectiveness of essential oils was discussed and, in most cases, confirmed. Now, it is time to determine whether their effectiveness can treat the symptoms of hormonal imbalances. While it is important to treat the symptoms, it is also crucial to understand and treat the cause. Yes, sometimes hormonal imbalances occur naturally in the body without reason and, in those cases, treating the symptoms is the only possible route. However, sometimes hormonal imbalances are brought about by external factors that may be within or outside of your control. For example, stress is a major influence and catalyst of hormonal imbalance. Extremely stressed people tend to have elevated levels of cortisol in their systems which, as you know, can result in weight gain, inflammation, and high blood pressure. In this instance, essential oils like clary sage, lavender, and rosemary can be an effective treatment of the symptoms caused by these imbalances. Not only do these oils have relaxing properties, but rosemary oil has been shown to lower the levels of cortisol present in saliva. Frankincense oil has anti-inflammatory properties and has been known to balance the hormones of the thyroid while also aiding in the soothing of menstrual cramps and mood swings. Peppermint oil is effective in treating the brain fog that accompanies so many different hormonal imbalances. If you suffer from forgetfulness, then rosemary oil can refresh your memory. Rose oil combats the many symptoms of testosterone imbalance and also helps with the sex drive.

Perhaps you have a poor diet, don't exercise much, and generally have an unhealthy lifestyle. Believe it or not, these factors can have a massive impact on hormone balance. Consuming too much alcohol or caffeine can affect cortisol and estrogen levels, leaving you vulnerable to an array of unpleasant hormonal imbalance symptoms. Eating unhealthily can increase your body's resistance to insulin which makes you susceptible to diabetes. In addition to using essential oils to cure the symptoms of hormonal imbalance, it is crucial to maintain a healthy and stable lifestyle. Think of your hormones like worker bees. It is way easier for the bees to pollinate flowers, travel back to the hive, and start making honey when they do not encounter obstacles. However, imagine the bee arriving at its favorite flower only to find it has already been pollinated. It goes to find another flower and collects some pollen. Suddenly, it gets stuck in some tree sap and struggles to get free. On the way back to the hive, the bee encounters several cars and birds until it finally arrives back at the hive. After this treacherous journey, the worker bee begins to make honey, except now it is a very tired worker bee and it struggles to maintain the same pace it once did. Similarly, if you throw obstacles in front of your hormones, like unhealthy eating habits, smoking, caffeine, and alcohol, your hormones and glands will have to work much harder to make up for the imbalanced lifestyle and will end up doing a mediocre job.

So, give your hormones a break. Make sure you are engaging in healthy lifestyle practices and remember that essential oils can help you on your journey to health and healing. Now that you know all about where essential oils came from, whether they work, how hormones work, and whether essential oils can contribute to their balancing, it is time to jump into the practical side of things.

Part 2:

A Holistic Exploration of What Essential Oils Can Do for You

Chapter 3

How to Use Essential Oils

There are many ways to use and apply essential oils. The method of application will often be defined by the hormonal imbalance that is being addressed. For example, digestive issues are best treated with a warm compress applied to the abdominal area. Some essential oils work best when consumed orally and others provide more relief when diffused or massaged into the skin. The best application methods for specific essential oils will be highlighted in-depth in the chapters concerning specific hormonal imbalances and their treatments. For now, it is important to have a basic understanding of the methods of application so that you can access the full potential of essential oils and their healing properties. While it is necessary to be aware of the different application methods for healing and treatment, it is also a matter of preference. Perhaps you enjoy using essential oils liberally and adding a few drops to your nighttime bath, perhaps you prefer to shower or find that dry evaporation is the best method for your busy life. There are no strict guidelines to follow and, whether you steam or diffuse, you will be reaping the benefits of essential oils. The journey to healing with essential oils is a holistic one. It is not linear or confining and can be explored with a sense of curiosity and acceptance.

Figure out what works for you and don't be afraid to experiment. Here are some of the most popular and effective essential oil application methods:

Mix with a Carrier Oil

Most essential oils will need to be mixed or diluted with another substance. This is because they are highly concentrated and can cause dryness or irritation of the skin. A popular way to dilute essential oils is to use a carrier oil. The carrier oil can be anything from jojoba oil to olive oil to coconut oil. This part of the process is rather subjective because you have to figure out which oil you like best and which one works well with your skin. It will take some trial and error but, once you have found the right carrier oil, you can add a few drops of the essential oil to the mix and massage it into your skin. You want the dilution ratio to be balanced, otherwise you could end up using too much carrier oil and lose out on the benefits of the essential oil. Alternatively, if too little of the carrier oil is added, you risk skin irritation. A good rule to follow is one drop of essential oil per teaspoon of carrier oil. Not only will this be gentle on the skin, but it will take the essential oil further so that you can use it for longer.

Mix with Cream

Similarly, to using a carrier oil, adding essential oils to cream, shampoo, conditioner, or any other soap you use regularly can benefit the body. When adding essential oils to cream, make sure that you are working with a relatively standard base. If the cream you are using already contains excessive amounts of additives, oils, and perfumes, it could overwhelm the skin and cause irritation. It is also important to be aware of your skin type when adding essential oils to face cream. If you have dry skin, you might want to avoid adding tea tree oil to the cream but, if you have oily skin, then using tea tree oil may be the right solution for you. Oils like lavender are also great for hair and can be added to shampoo and conditioner. Following the same rationale with a carrier oil (one drop per one teaspoon) will allow you to adequately dilute the essential oil. However, it might be difficult to measure a pot of face cream in teaspoons. In that case, follow the ratio of two to four drops per ounce.

Diffuse

Diffusing essential oils is a great way to experience the healing powers of essential oils without actually doing anything. If you have a nebulizer or a water diffuser, you just add a few drops and the diffuser will do the rest. Along with releasing the healing scents of these oils, it can also help to purify the air in your house. Unfortunately, due to rising pollution, the air is often polluted and toxic. Using essential oils to create a haven from this pollution might be just what you need to fight off the rising levels of carbon dioxide in the earth's atmosphere. However, while using a diffuser is easy and you might be tempted to leave it on the whole day—don't. Use it daily and leave it on for an hour, at most. Excessive exposure to essential oils can lead to headaches and other adverse symptoms. Moderation is key when it comes to using essential oils.

Add to Bath/Shower

As with using cream and a carrier oil to dilute the essential oil, it is also useful to add a few drops of essential oils to a bath. Depending on the size of the bath and the amount of water, a good amount would be anywhere between 10 and 20 drops. If you prefer showering, splash a few drops onto the walls of the shower. The steam from the water will activate the essential oil and allow you to reap the benefits of a full-body essential oil steam. Similarly, the steam from a bath will carry the oils up to your nose and mouth and allow you to inhale the essential oils while absorbing them into your body through the water. This method is perfect for reducing stress and muscle pain.

Dry Evaporation

This method is perfect for anyone who is always on-the-go and rarely has a moment to themselves. If you find that you are rushed and stressed, moving between meetings, rushing to pick up children, and unable to take a minute for yourself, then dry evaporation is the perfect essential oil application method for you. Place a few drops onto a cotton ball and hold it up to your nose. The cotton ball can also be placed near you, like on a desk or in the car. Take a few deep breaths for instant relief from hormonal imbalance symptoms. Try not to inhale for too long as the cotton ball contains pure, concentrated essential oil which can be quite potent.

Steaming

Similar to diffusion and using essential oils in a bath or shower, targeted steaming is a great way to inhale essential oils without applying them directly to the skin. Pour hot water (hot enough to produce steam) into a bowl that is large enough to cover your whole face. Add five to ten drops of essential oil into the water, place a towel over your head, and proceed to inhale the steam. Try to do this in intervals of one to two minutes as too much exposure to essential oils can have adverse effects. Once you have steamed, don't just throw away the water, use it to mop floors or clean surfaces. Remember, essential oils have antibacterial qualities and can benefit you in all aspects of your life. Steaming is also a great way to help with illness. The essential oils and steam work to clear out the nasal and respiratory tracts for easier breathing. The antibacterial and antifungal qualities of essential oils also help to fight off bacteria caused by illness.

Linen/Room Spray

This method is perfect for a little rush of essential oil magic. To make linen spray, all you need is alcohol (preferably vodka as it is scentless), water, and a few drops of an essential oil of your choice (preferably one that induces sleep, like lavender oil). Mix the ingredients and add to a spray bottle. Spray onto the bed a few minutes before you get in and enjoy a peaceful night's rest. Due to the low concentration of essential oil and the fact that the material absorbs the mixture relatively quickly, the smell will disappear within a few hours so you don't have to worry about inhaling too much of the essential oil mixture. A room spray can be made in the same way, except you might want to swap out the lavender oil with lemongrass or orange oil to provide a fresh citrus scent. Spray into the room whenever you need for a pick-me-up or mood boost.

Orally

It is important to note that not all essential oils can be ingested. In fact, very few oils can be ingested. These include cassia, lemon, cinnamon, thyme, clove, oregano, lime, grapefruit, peppermint. There are many more but ingesting essential oils always comes with some degree of risk. Because most essential oils are unregulated, it can be dangerous to consume them. Ingesting essential oils should therefore be approached with caution. If you want to consume them orally you can add a few drops to a smoothie or drinking water, but a drop or two will be sufficient. If possible, oral ingestion should be avoided but if administered appropriately and alongside a herbalist or medical professional, the oral ingestion of essential oils can be beneficial to healing and hormone balance. However, the point of essential oil therapy and aromatherapy is to benefit from the scent of the oil, which is not possible if ingested. Also, the body can absorb these oils when applied to the skin and it is not necessary to ingest them to be able to benefit from the oils. Therefore, administering essential oils orally is not typically advised.

Targeted Application

This particular method works if you want to target a specific area of the body. For example, tea tree oil has been proven to cure acne and, in this case, applying tea tree oil (that is diluted with a cream or carrier oil) to the affected areas on the face can be used to treat acne. Additionally, there are several oils, like peppermint and calendula oil, that can help with eczema. Targeted application to affected areas can speed up the healing process and provide relief from symptoms of hormonal imbalance.

Warm Compress

This method helps with headaches, stomach pains, and any kind of internal or external inflammation. If you are feeling bloated or suffering from cramps, you can soak a small towel in water and a few drops of essential oils. Place the compress on the affected area for relief from swelling, inflammation, and pain. The heat from the compress can help soothe aches and also releases the essential oil aroma. It is similar to steaming except with an element of targeted application as the warm compress is applied specifically to areas of pain and inflammation.

Safety First

Just because essential oils come from nature does not mean that they do not carry harmful side-effects when used recklessly or improperly. To make use of their full potential, essential oils must be used appropriately. Similarly to how your body may react to an excess or deficit in hormone production, your body can react to too much and too little essential oils. Here are a few important steps to practice when using essential oils:

Patch Test

While you might like to think that you know your body, sometimes skin, tissues, and muscles can react in unexpected ways. This is why it is important to do a patch test. A patch test is a test to determine whether you have any kind of reaction or aversion to the specific oil being used. Before adding essential oils to all of your cream, oil, and shampoo, make sure to dilute some with a carrier oil and test it on a small piece of skin. The underside of the wrist provides a good indication of whether your skin will have an adverse reaction to the essential oil. Besides, you don't want to discover that you may be allergic to lavender oil after you have added it to every cream you own. Approach essential oils with caution, test the waters, and make sure your journey to healing is as smooth as possible.

Make Sure the Oil Is Produced by a Reliable Supplier

It might be easier to figure out which pharmaceutical medicine is best for you because they are regulated by the FDA (Food and Drug Administration). Unfortunately, essential oils are not regulated by the FDA, so it is a little more challenging to spot the fakes. To make the process easier, there are a few things to look out for. First, the essential oil bottle must be dark and made from glass. Some essential oils can dissolve plastic. If the essential oil comes in a plastic bottle, it is a clear indication that the oil is either heavily diluted or merely a fragrance. If the bottle says "essence oil" or "fragrance oil," it is not an essential oil. The information on the bottle must include the plant name, the Latin plant name, the plant material used in processing, and the method of extraction. All of this information will allow you to sift out the authentic essential oils from the fakes. Also, the bottle should mention somewhere that it is

"100% pure essential oil." If all of these requisites are confirmed, then you can give that supplier the green light.

Do Not Ingest Unless Otherwise Advised

Ingesting tea tree, eucalyptus, and wintergreen oil have particularly adverse effects on the body. Ingesting these oils could result in vomiting, increased heart rate, and even kidney damage. Realistically, it is better not to ingest any essential oils, but if you must, it is best to avoid those just mentioned oils. Also, if the patch test caused an allergic reaction, then ingesting the oil will likely have the same effect.

Do Not Inhale for Extended Periods

While you might be enjoying the world of essential oils and you just want to smell them all the time, this probably isn't such a great idea. Prolonged inhalation of essential oils can lead to headaches, increased heart rate, and increased blood pressure. Moderation is the name of the game. You shouldn't be rubbing essential oils onto your body twice a day while allowing steam from the diffuser to engulf your house. Stick to two 30-minute sessions a day and use the cream once a day. While you may not be able to overdose on essential oils as you can with certain pharmaceutical drugs, it is still necessary to practice restraint for the best results.

Consult Your Doctor

This step is crucial, especially if using essential oil and aromatherapy as a supplementary treatment to any medication you might already be taking. While doctors probably won't dissuade you from using essential oils, they can give you advice on how to use them to compliment your specific hormonal imbalance or condition. It is also important to be aware of any allergies or aversions you might have to essential oils. Remember, essential oils don't claim to be as effective as pharmaceutical treatments, however, they do provide holistic healing and can benefit most treatment plans and medicines.

Do Not Use Undiluted Essential Oils

As previously mentioned, essential oils are highly concentrated extracts derived from plant material. This means that they have the power to cause irritation, itching, and even burns on the skin. Similarly to how fruit juice concentrate contains a lot more sugar than fruit juice and can be harmful to your body if drunk in excess, essential oils can do the same (if not worse). So, figure out your favorite method of dilution, be it using a cream or carrier oil, and make sure the ratios are optimal.

Watch out for Sensitive Areas of the Body

Using undiluted essential oils can be harmful on any and all parts of the body, but using diluted essential oils in sensitive areas can be just as harmful. Stay away from the mouth, eyes, and pubic regions of the body to avoid irritation, swelling, and burning. Unless otherwise advised, these areas should always be avoided.

Storage

This is one of the most important steps in using essential oils because if they are not stored properly, they can quickly become rancid without your knowledge. Firstly, the bottle must be glass and dark in color because light and heat can alter the chemical balance of the essential oils. This also means the bottle should be stored in a cool, dark, and dry place, like a cupboard. The lid must be airtight because exposure to air activates the properties of the essential oil. The longer they are left open or exposed to air the less concentrated the oils will be. Make sure the essential oils are kept at a constant temperature as shifts in temperature can also cause disturbances in the chemical balance of the oils.

Tips and Tricks for Using Essential Oils

Essential Oils Can Expire

Yes, unfortunately, essential oils can expire—another reason why choosing the right supplier is so crucial. The right supplier will ensure that all containers are airtight, uncontaminated, and usable for at least 12 months. Practicing the proper storage techniques will also ensure that your essential oils last longer. It is important to be aware of the expiration date of the essential oil because using rancid and expired oils can be ineffective or lead to skin irritation and burning. If you still have half a bottle left and the oil expires next week, fear not! There are many fun and exciting ways to use up essential oils before they turn rancid. For example, using them to make bath salts. Salt acts as a natural preservative and can be used for baths and as gifts. Using the leftover oils to make candles is also an option. So, don't just throw the oils away in defeat. They still have so much to offer.

Reuse Empty Bottles

Just like you shouldn't be throwing away the essential oils, you shouldn't be throwing away the bottles, either. These are perfect little containers for travel size, pre-diluted essential oils so that you can have access to them wherever you go. Put a few in your car, at work, in the kitchen, give some to your children or your partner. Because using essential oils is a holistic form of healing, it is pertinent that the whole process is considered. Living in a polluted and wasteful society is not conducive to healing and playing your part in reducing this waste is also part of the path to healing.

Keep Age in Mind

You might want everyone to join in on the buzz. However, it is important to note that age does affect the amount of essential oils one should be taking in. As a child, the recommended dosage is half of the dosage for an adult (which is one drop per one teaspoon). The same goes for pregnant women. During these stages of life, children and pregnant women are generally more sensitive to stimuli. Using highly concentrated oils may be too intense for these groups of people; therefore, a lower dosage is recommended.

Use It in Modeling Clay

Just because children require a smaller dosage of essential oils does not mean that they can't still have fun. Putting a few drops of essential oil into homemade or store-bought modeling clay can bring about hours of fun with a healthy dose of essential oil goodness. Using modeling clay is effective in several ways; mainly, if children are experiencing flu symptoms or nasal congestion, this is a fun way to help clear up those airways. Depending on which essential oil you put into the modeling clay, the antibacterial and antifungal properties of some oils can be an easy way to ensure that your kids aren't playing with a giant ball of bacteria. It keeps the modeling clay clean and smells great.

Use It to Disinfect Surfaces

Similarly to how essential oils can help to disinfect modeling clay, they can also clean the surfaces of toys, countertops, floors, bathrooms, and car interiors, and clothes. Add a few drops to detergent or other cleaning mediums to leave spaces clean, free of bacteria, and smelling good. Not only will it work to clean your house but you can also reap the benefits of inhaling the oils.

Candles/Incense

Candles and incense can also be used as an additional aromatherapy. Try to buy candles that are made from natural ingredients, like beeswax, and have natural aromas. While a strawberry-scented candle might smell amazing, it probably won't provide any health benefits. Instead, go for a frankincense or jasmine scented candle to mimic the healing effects of frankincense or jasmine oil. Incense sticks can also be effective for aromatherapy purposes. Incense is made out of wood, resins, tree gum, and aromatics to give off an earthy and spicy scent. In this case, it is also best to choose a scent that is in line with essential oils, like cinnamon, frankincense, sandalwood, or patchouli. Using these scents will allow you to reap some of the benefits of essential oil therapy while trying out a different medium.

Essential Oils Can Boost Your Immune System

Not only can they cure illness and alleviate the symptoms of illness but they can also prevent it. Using essential oils preventatively can stop you from succumbing to those pesky winter colds. The best essential oils to use for immune-boosting purposes are lemon, clary sage, lavender, rosemary, clove, thyme, peppermint, tea tree, and chamomile oil because they inhibit the growth of bacteria, and have relaxing and clearing properties that help to prevent illness.

How to Massage Oil into the Skin

There are four key areas on the body which can benefit from essential oil absorption. The choice of area depends on your preference and which hormonal imbalance or condition you are treating. These areas include:

- Head: The diluted essential oil can be rubbed into the temples (the sides of the head) and in the middle of the forehead, between the eyebrows. These are known as pressure points and can promote relaxation. The oil is also in close proximity to the face and, therefore, allows the benefits of aromatherapy to be experienced.

- Wrists: Along with the temples and middle of the forehead, wrists are also pressure points and can be gently massaged as the essential oil is absorbed into the skin.
- Feet: Using the practice of reflexology (medical massaging of the feet and hands) essential oils can work in unison with the healing properties of reflexology. Additionally, if you experience odor or foot fungus, the essential oil can mask the smell and treat the fungus.
- Chest: Gently rubbing the essential oil solution onto the chest can clear and open up the chest from illness or tension.

These areas can be gently massaged in a circular motion to effectively spread the essential oil solution onto the skin for maximum absorption.

There are so many exciting, unique, and useful ways to use essential oils to help you in your journey to healing and hormone balance. Maybe inspiration strikes and you make a linen spray for your towels or you decide to add some scented candles to the mix. Once you start on the essential oil train, there is no stopping. So, get creative, enjoy the process, and start incorporating essential oils into your daily life. Just remember to stay safe, store them appropriately, and never apply them to the skin undiluted. Now that you know what to watch out for, it is time to understand how essential oils can contribute to the holistic healing of your mind, body, and soul.

Chapter 4

How Essential Oils Can Help You Mentally, Spiritually, and Physically

The list of advantages to using essential oils feels like it could go on forever. If they aren't helping you to feel relaxed, they are making your skin look great or soothing the symptoms of hormonal imbalance. There are so many innovative and exciting ways to incorporate essential oils into your daily life. But before you do, it is useful to know how essential oils can send you on a journey to fulfilment and holistic healing. Pharmaceutical medicine often serves one purpose. If you take a headache pill, it will help with your headache. If you take medication for indigestion, it will soothe your stomach. However, these medicines rarely have any other advantages. Plus, you end up taking several different pills for all of your ailments instead of using just one or two essential oils. Not only that, but essential oils provide a holistic and gentle path to healing. Instead of targeting one specific area, they can help you to find relief mentally, spiritually, and physically.

Mentally

One of the ways that essential oils and aromatherapy can help is by improving mental health. The world is a busy and chaotic place, even without the extra weight of maintaining people's expectations, surviving on minimum wage, and trying to live up to the high standards you have set for yourself. Try as you might, it always feels like somewhere, someone is disappointed in you. You rush from meeting to meeting, errand to errand, as you try to run away from the overwhelming feelings of anxiety and depression. Luckily, it can be easy to outrun those feelings when you are busy and preoccupied. However, when you have a quiet moment, you might wonder why you still feel rushed and antsy. Well, it's no wonder you might be feeling that way. While pharmaceutical medicines also have their place in treating mental health, so do essential oils.

Many essential oils, like lavender, cedarwood, and jasmine, have calming properties. These oils can help to calm a busy mind. Whether you are struggling to sleep or just need to refocus your mind to the present, essential oils can ease the symptoms of anxiety so that you can function in everyday life. Applying essential oils diluted in carrier oil or cream to the temples and forehead is a great way to get a healthy dose of calm straight to your brain. It is also worth noting that humans carry stress in different places. You might carry stress in your jaw, neck, shoulders, or arms. Use essential oils to target and massage these specific areas for added relief.

Essential oils are also effective in treating symptoms of depression. Depression comes in many different shapes and sizes and each individual's experience is different. If you find that your depression makes you feel exhausted and unable to complete tasks, try using lemon or grapefruit oil. These oils have energizing properties and may provide relief from fatigue. As I said at the beginning of this book, essential oils are not going to heal your trauma, but they can relieve the symptoms so that you can live a better and healthier life. Depending on how you experience depression and what your symptoms might be, find an oil that addresses your specific situation. Perhaps using a calming oil, like lavender, will only put you to sleep, and this won't be useful if you have already slept through most of the day. Treating the symptoms of anxiety and depression is about creating enough space for you to deal with the causes of the mental illnesses. If you are constantly tired and sleeping, then dealing with and treating depression is nearly impossible. However, using essential oils to provide a small hit of energy can give you the strength to start addressing the causes and catalysts of the mental health disorder.

Perhaps you don't struggle with depression or anxiety but suffer from mood swings. Essential oils are natural mood stabilizers and can be used to bring your mood back to equilibrium. Even if you are simply having a bad day, a whiff of lavender oil can put you back on track in an instant. It's kind of like when you come home to the smell of freshly baked cookies. No matter how awful your day or how busy you are, that smell takes you back to a happier time. Suddenly, you are no longer thinking of the deadline you have to meet tomorrow, but are preoccupied with the thought of dunking that steaming hot cookie into a glass of cold milk. While certain oils have specific calming or energizing properties, find an essential oil that brings you joy and use it as a tool for getting through those tough days.

If you struggle with insomnia or restlessness, lavender and chamomile oil have soothing and relaxing properties that allow your brain to slow down and rest. No more long nights spent tossing and turning, thinking about the fight you had with someone from grade school. No more tired mornings steeped in coffee so you can make it through the day. Placing a warm compress on the forehead or using a linen spray is a great way to treat insomnia. The warmth and gentle lavender scent will put you to sleep in no time.

On top of helping with mental health, essential oils can also promote a healthy mindset. It is easy to get bogged down by all the horrible things happening in the world. However, our lives and minds don't need to become engulfed and consumed by this negativity. Essential oils can bring back some joy into your life. Along with the practices of mindfulness and gratitude, the holistic nature of essential oils can lift you out of the stream of negativity and allow you to see and notice the joy of existence. Treating and alleviating the symptoms of anxiety, depression, and fear can give you the time and space to notice the world around you in a positive light. Using essential oils will also leave you feeling rejuvenated, motivated, and ready to take on the day.

Spiritually

Essential oils have a way of bringing you back to reality. In the next chapter, I will highlight the importance of practicing mindfulness and presence in conjunction with using essential oils. While practicing mindfulness and using essential oils to promote spiritual healing and different practices, they should not be seen as two separate philosophies. The process of using or applying an essential oil means that you are focusing on one moment, one task, and one scent. Your brain is not preoccupied with what you still have to do today or how much work you have. Also, merely being aware of the scent that the essential oil produces can ground you back in reality and stop your mind from wandering too far into the past or future. The application process, along with the active awareness of the scent, can bring you back to yourself and allow you to practice mindfulness and presence more effectively and holistically.

Many ancient cultures used essential oils in their religions. The ancient Egyptians used perfumes and oils to honor and pay respect to the gods. They also valued scent and smelling nice and included essential oils in the mummification process not only for their antibacterial properties but so that the dead could ascend into the afterlife and meet the gods with a pleasant scent. In Ayurveda, essential oils are used to create a holistic balance between mind, body, and soul. Throughout history, essential oils have not only been used for their healing properties but were, and still are, central parts of religious practice and spiritual guidance.

Essential oils can be cleansing not only for the body but for the mind and soul. By allowing you to see the joy of life and creating a space for you to function without the symptoms of stress and anxiety or other conditions, they give your heart and soul the space to gain an understanding of life. By removing pain, weakness, fatigue, and mental illness from your life, you can reach an equilibrium between the mind, body, and soul and nourish these aspects of the self. Instead of worrying about what to make for dinner or impressing your new boss by working overtime, use this time and energy to discover yourself. Figure out what makes you tick. Analyze your actions, figure out how and who you want to be, and release the negative forces within you. Essential oils can help with more than just hormonal imbalances.

Spiritual growth is about transcending worldly boundaries. It might sound impossible because, after all, you live on this planet, you have a human form, and you have to function as an active member of society. While all of this is true, spiritual growth is still possible. Growing spiritually means finding your place in existence—finding your purpose, if you will. It is about self-analyzing and self-actualizing so that you can be the best version of yourself possible. If you are constantly living in the past or the future, then this healing and growth can never happen. However, we all have our good and bad weeks. Sometimes everything is progressing and you feel confident and motivated and then, suddenly, a slump hits. You are riddled with self-doubt and frustration. Nothing seems to be going right and spiritual growth is just not on the table. Essential oils can get you back to where you need to be. By refocusing and taking care of yourself, a whiff of rose oil may be just the thing you need.

The process of administering essential oils and allowing yourself to engage with aromatherapy can also be a way of showing up for yourself. Sometimes, instead of taking care of everyone else and their needs, all you need to do is practice some self-care to show yourself that you are important and deserve to be healthy and balanced. Take a few moments out of the day to take a long bath, or meditate while the diffuser wafts essential oils in your direction. Either way, taking a moment for yourself will clear up negative pathways and allow you to approach life with a sense of openness.

Physically

Mental and spiritual healing, while different, are in a similar realm. The physical realm is more tangible. If something hurts, you can point to it. Contrastingly, you can't point to a specific part of the body to treat depression and you can't quantify spiritual growth and healing. However, in the physical realm, it is easier to do this. It is easier to identify hormonal imbalances, pain, and scarring. So how can essential oils help you in the physical realm?

For starters, if you have a wound, you can use essential oils to disinfect, clean, and heal it. Due to the antibacterial and antifungal properties of some essential oils, they can be applied to an open wound to prevent infection. In addition to inhibiting the growth of bacteria, essential oils also speed up the rate of healing. Some oils, like tea tree oil, dry out the skin and can be effective in combating oily skin. However, in the case of burns, tea tree oil will not be effective as burns require moisture to heal. Lavender oil will be more successful in treating the burn. However, when treating open wounds, the drying qualities of tea tree oil can speed up healing and leave your skin unblemished in no time.

Tea tree oil is also used for the treatment of acne for the very same reason. Essential oils not only clear up but rejuvenate skin, giving it a glowing appearance. Lavender oil nourishes skin and leaves it looking clean and fresh while frankincense oil evens out complexion and helps with dark circles under the eyes. If you require some moisture, clary sage oil can moisturize your skin and soothe any irritations.

Not only do essential oils make your skin feel great, they can also revitalize hair. Peppermint oil can activate the hair follicles and stimulate blood flow through the scalp, thus promoting hair growth. So if you want to grow your hair, peppermint oil should be the go-to option. Lemongrass oil nourishes the scalp and reduces dandruff.

While essential oils nourish and repair the outside of your body, they can also correct imbalances inside of your body. The healing effects of essential oils on hormonal imbalance can be life changing. For example, jasmine oil has aphrodisiac properties and can be used to increase sex drive. Alternatively, grapefruit oil can help to lower blood pressure. Each oil has a specific purpose that can be tailored to your needs.

Essential oils can help with aches and pains, as well as muscle soreness. After you exercise, a warm compress with chamomile can be applied to the sore muscles. Chamomile oil has anti-inflammatory properties that can reduce swelling or general stiffness. Warm compresses can also be applied to areas to alleviate the pain of headaches and stomachaches.

When essential oils are incorporated into your life, you will immediately be able to tell the difference, not only in your mental state, but in your body and soul. You will be able to float through life and take on any obstacles in your way with quiet confidence. Feeling stressed? Try a warm compress with a few drops of frankincense oil. Feeling tired? Orange oil will perk you right up. However, seeing as essential oil therapy is a holistic treatment and journey, there are a few practices you can include in your lifestyle that will optimize the effects of essential oils on your journey to healing.

Chapter 5

Practices That Aid in the Effectiveness of Essential Oils

Essential oils are useful when used independently; however, because they form part of holistic healing, one of the main focuses of essential oil therapy is to bring balance. To live a balanced life means to be conscious of your mind, body, and soul as a whole system of being and not just three aspects of human life. To get the most out of essential oils and aromatherapy, other aspects of life must also be balanced. If you are stuck in a negative mindset, refuse to make goals, don't take time to reflect, and live a generally unhealthy lifestyle, then essential oils will help you—but not successfully. While living an unbalanced life is not ideal and the benefits of essential oils will be reduced, they can open up the possibility of balancing your life in all aspects of being. As you reach mental, spiritual, and physical equilibrium, you will be able to notice the full effects of essential oil therapy. Here are a few practices to get you started:

Mentally

Positive Thinking

Positive thinking does not mean you have to ignore everything negative and forget that bad things happen. Positive thinking is about maintaining an uplifted and grateful attitude, despite the negative things happening around you. For example, say you go on holiday to a tropical island and, the whole time you are there, it is storming and thundering. You can't go to the beach, you can't walk around the island, and every fun activity has been shut down. Instead, you have to stay indoors, order room service, and watch your holiday crash and burn. There are two options. You could either stay in your room for the rest of the holiday, miserable and alone, and leave a day early because you can't bear to watch the remnants of your holiday get washed away by the rain. Or, you could maintain a positive attitude, despite the outcome of your holiday, go down to the lobby, and meet a few interesting travelers. You can decide to stay for the entirety of the holiday. In this version of the story, the sky clears up, the ocean is crystal clear, and you have a few new friends with whom to go snorkeling. Indulging negative thoughts, in this situation, would get you nowhere. You wouldn't have met anyone new, you wouldn't get to enjoy the most beautiful day of your holiday, and you would have spent the next few months feeling sorry for yourself. However, when maintaining a positive attitude, opportunity presents itself.

Similarly, if you go through life with a negative mindset, essential oils will only be able to help you to a certain degree. While it is natural to be skeptical, and one should be aware of the dangers of certain treatments, the effectiveness of essential oil therapy can be reduced if you don't believe in the healing powers of aromatherapy. Think of Peter Pan and Tinkerbell. When the characters said they didn't believe in fairies, Tinkerbell started to lose her life force. She was no longer able to fly or help anyone. But, as soon as they started chanting, *I do believe in fairies*, she came back to life. Understandably, fairies and essential oils are not comparable. However, the power of positive thinking remains at the core of this comparison. If you fill your mind with negative thoughts, like *essential oils won't work* or *I'm never going to get better*, then essential oils probably won't work as well for you and you might not get better. Picture negative thoughts as closed doors. How can healing begin if it can't even gain access to the mind, body, and soul? Positive thoughts are wide open doors ready to embrace the possibilities and unpredictability of life. Unfortunately, bad things happen and they happen to everyone. There is no doubt that you will have to deal with unpleasantness or heartache. But, while you may not have any control over the events that occur in your life, you do have control over how you react to them.

The practice of gratitude is one of the most effective ways to maintain a positive attitude. While it might feel like there is no upside to the negative things happening to and around you, there is always a positive way of looking at a situation. Instead of falling into a depressive cycle of negative thoughts because you lost your job, be grateful that you now have the opportunity to explore other interests and career opportunities. Instead of worrying about the cost of repairs on your car, be grateful that you have a car. Practicing gratitude will not only show you that you have a lot for which to be thankful but will allow you to see the silver lining in every situation.

Another useful technique to maintain positive thinking is using positive mantras. These can either be highly specific to your situation or more general. Repeat these phrases on a daily basis and whenever you are experiencing negative thoughts. Possible phrases may include:

1. *I am successful*
2. *I am worthy of living a healthy lifestyle and taking care of myself*
3. *I am going to heal*

Whichever mantra you choose, make sure it motivates you to continue working towards your goals and helps you to maintain a positive mental attitude.

Creative Visualization

Creative visualization takes positive thinking a step further. It does not only require you to think positively, but to imagine the possibility of success, healing, happiness, health, and whatever else you desire. For creative visualization, you must have a set of goals. For example, you may want to heal a hormonal imbalance or chronic pain. The process of creative visualization involves imagination and is a marriage between meditation and positive thinking. For this process to be successful, you need goals, structure, and time. The goals are essential because they will form part of the visualization process. Structure is required to train your brain and make sure you are actively participating in the process. Set up a schedule that incorporates the various facets of your lifestyle, as well as your preferences. If you like to wake up early in the morning, start a ritual whereby you make some coffee, water the plants, and find a cozy space to begin the visualization process. Set aside time from your day to practice creative visualization. This can be anywhere from 10 minutes to an hour. However, for the practice to be successful, you have to use the dedicated time without any distractions, worries, or plans.

Once the goals, structure, and time elements of the practice have been identified and planned out, it is time to begin visualization. The first step is to close your eyes. Close them for a few minutes and try to embrace the quiet and stillness before beginning the visualization. Get comfortable with the darkness. Then, instead of projecting your visualization onto the back of your eyelids, picture a giant screen that fills the sky. So giant you can almost not see where it ends and begins. Then, start the movie. If one of your goals is to heal the symptoms of insomnia with essential oils, then there are two routes to visualization. The first route is picturing the process. Picture yourself inhaling, diffusing, or applying the essential oil. If you picture diffusing, then imagine the scent particles from the essential oils flowing into your nose and activating the neurons and smell receptors. Picture the neurons sending messages to your brain and body to relax the muscles, close the eyes, and drift into a comfortable slumber. Don't just stop there! Picture the softness of your pillow. Imagine the feeling of the sheets against your body, the heaviness of your limbs. Creative visualization is about using all five senses to create a full and seemingly real visual. The second route is to picture your life without insomnia. Visualize how you might feel with a good night's rest. Are you energetic? Picture waking up in the morning, jumping out of bed excited and ready to take on the day. Maybe you engage in a yoga practice or take a run down to the coffee shop to eat breakfast. Visualize how the breakfast tastes, how you feel and what a life without insomnia might look like.

While it may take a few times to get into the swing of things, creative visualization is a great way to maintain positive thinking. It also promotes self-reflection and helps you to achieve your goals. Wondering how it works? Well, whether you are thinking of lifting your arm or are actually lifting your arm, the same neurons are activated in the brain. Therefore, when you are thinking about healing and getting better, those same neurons that help you heal are being used. It has been scientifically shown to help athletes reach greater heights and speeds. Patients who were once terminally ill used creative visualization to heal and live a life they never imagined. While it is not guaranteed that creative visualization will turn you into an Olympic athlete or cure you of an incurable disease, the benefits of this practice are still noteworthy.

Spiritually

Meditation

Similarly to creative visualization, meditation can also help maintain a positive mindset, although it is not quite as active as creative visualization. It might feel intimidating at first, especially if you hear stories about people who can meditate anywhere, for any amount of time. You don't have to be a grandmaster to be able to reap the benefits of meditation. To start, your practice can last for as little as three minutes until you work your way up to 15 and 30-minute sessions.

But, how do I meditate? You might be wondering. There are several methods of meditation. One method is known as movement meditation. This can be practiced while walking or creating small movements with the body. It aims to engage the body and mind while bringing stillness to the mind and spirit. Focused meditation is similar to creative visualization as it involves entering the meditation with a specific purpose or goal in mind. It also uses all five senses to ground the body and mind while uplifting the spirit. Then, there is mindfulness meditation which is the most widely practiced form of meditation. It involves clearing the mind for a certain period of time to achieve enlightenment. I know, enlightenment is a tall order, but give it a chance and you will see how a few moments of quiet reflection and the scent of essential oils can bring you back into yourself.

As for how to meditate, you start by closing your eyes. You can either employ breathing techniques or you can focus on the natural rhythm of your breath. In terms of breathing techniques, you can breathe in for 10 seconds, and out for 10 seconds (or any amount of time you are comfortable with). Practice breathing in through the nose and out through the mouth and even try alternating nostrils by holding one closed as you breathe in and alternating on the next breath. Breathing techniques are useful in the beginning when being conscious about your breath may feel awkward and forced. Once you have mastered a few breathing techniques, follow the natural rhythm of your breath. Try not to focus on anything else. If your mind wanders, bring it back to your breath. Focus on how it affects your body. Does your belly inflate? Feel the air fill your lungs and your ribcage expand and contract as you breathe in and out. It is kind of like being in a trance. Nothing else exists except you and your breath.

Meditation can help to lower heart rate, blood pressure, and cortisol levels. This practice works well alone and together with essential oils. You can diffuse essential oils into the room while you meditate. This will not only help to relax you but it can aid in the grounding process (a central facet of meditation). Incorporating meditation into your daily life, like positive thinking, will open doors for essential oil therapy to work to its full potential.

Mindfulness

Meditation and mindfulness go hand-in-hand because these practices work to ground you and bring you into the present moment. Have you ever tried to go to sleep and find that there are thousands of little thoughts running through your mind? Suddenly, a cringey memory from middle school appears and you obsess over how you acted and what you could have changed. Then, it transforms into worries about your future and how you don't know where your life is going. In the midst of all of these thoughts, it's almost like you forgot that you exist. You live in the past and future now and the present moment has no influence over you. Did you ever think about what it feels like to exist while you were having those intrusive thoughts and memories? Are you conscious of the texture of the pillow, the breath moving through your body, the feeling of your body in a specific time, the slight glow from the street light into your dark room. Maybe it is easy to get lost in those moments because there is nothing else to think about. But are you present in other moments of your life? Are you present at a dinner party with your friends or does your mind wander to deadlines and meetings? What do you do when you are sitting at the dinner table 10 years later wondering where your life has gone? Wondering how you spent your time and what you did. Not being present can cause you to slide through life without any intention or thought until one day you wonder how you got to where you are.

Mindfulness is about bringing awareness to the body, mind, and soul in the exact moment you are in. It is about being intentional with your thoughts, actions, and feelings. Using essential oils can bring you back into the present moment and stop you from time travelling to the past or future because those are time frames in which you have no control. At least, you have no control over the past. However, despite the lack of control over the past, it is still important to learn from it. That is why practicing presence and intentionality are important because intentionality allows you to think about your actions and presence forces you not to obsess over them.

Practicing mindfulness is similar to meditation except mindfulness will eventually become a way of life and not merely a practice. Mindfulness can and should be implemented at every point in your day, whether you are working, cooking, eating, or sleeping. It can help you to stay focused and motivated. To practice mindfulness, you should bring awareness to your body, to the feeling of existing in that exact moment. Start by bringing awareness to your toes. Concentrate on how they feel, the pressure on the bottom of your foot as you stand, feel them tingle with energy as you move up the body to bring awareness to your feet, legs, knees, thighs, stomach, shoulders, arms, neck, and head, until your entire body is tingling with awareness. This can be done with open or closed eyes, as long as you concentrate on what it means to be alive in the present moment. This may take some practice but reminding yourself to stay focused on the present will pay off in the end. Instead of wondering where your life has gone, you will be able to treasure the moments and memories in which you were present and active.

Physically

Eating Healthily

For the same reasons you may be looking at using essential oils as a treatment therapy, eating healthy and nutritious food can provide you with some of the nutrients your body needs to function. Eating fruits, vegetables, and grains is a great way to restore balance within the body. There are many diets and fasting techniques available at the moment. Some of them are not effective or healthy, and others may only work for certain people. At the end of the day, you shouldn't starve yourself to get to a goal weight or stress eat because it makes you feel better. Having a healthy relationship with food will help you change the way you view your body. It is not a vessel with the sole purpose of looking a certain way and it is also not a disposable machine that you can disregard. Your body is a living organism made up of millions of different nerve endings, neurons, hormones, and cells that work extremely hard to keep you alive. You don't like your arms? Well, they can help you pick things up and drive and, without them, life would be more difficult. Being grateful for your body and all of the things it does for you makes eating healthily an act of self-care.

Now, everyone is different. People have different preferences, likes and dislikes, allergies, and requirements and creating a universal diet for you to live by is actually quite unrealistic. Therefore, instead of providing you with a dietary plan or a calorie-counting fasting schedule, I will leave you with this: Eating healthy is about balance. If your diet consists of 90% red meat and 10% carbohydrates, your diet is not balanced, nor is it very healthy. To practice eating a healthy and balanced diet, make sure you have an equal amount of protein, grains, carbohydrates, minerals, and vitamins in your diet. As I said, everyone is different and you may want to increase the number of vegetables in relation to carbohydrates or vice versa. As long as there is a semblance of balance and your body is getting everything it needs you can structure the diet in a way that suits and excites you.

Remember, everything in moderation. Being aware of your body and what it needs is the best way to ensure you are living a healthy lifestyle. The body needs a certain amount of sugar to function and depriving the body can lead to harmful repercussions. Make sure you are eating fruits and vegetables, be sure to control portion sizes, and don't be afraid to treat yourself every once in a while. However, try to stay away from fast food, junk food, and any other synthetically produced foods as they can contribute to hormonal imbalance.

Exercise

To bring balance to your mind and soul, your body needs to be engaged. Holistic healing does not mean you can pick and choose which parts of yourself that you want to heal. It is about healing and bringing balance to the entire being. Not only does exercising open your body and mind up through stretching and strengthening. It also gets your heart rate going, lowers blood pressure, and releases dopamine and serotonin into the body. Remember those amazing hormones? Those are the hormones that make you feel happy, and if you feel happy, positive thinking and creative visualization become easier and way more fulfilling.

Similarly to eating healthily, people are different and prefer different methods of exercising. If you don't like jogging, don't torture yourself. Try swimming or walking, instead. Perhaps you enjoy going to the gym or cycling in your neighborhood. Whichever form of exercise you enjoy and works well with your body and schedule is not only going to make you happy, but it will play a positive role in bringing balance to your mind, body, and soul.

Unlike meditation and mindfulness, you don't have to exercise every single day to be balanced. Use a system that works for you and go from there. Perhaps you are not used to a regular exercising schedule and want to start slow. All you need is one day a week, one 30-minute session to get yourself excited and motivated. Increase the sessions as you gain confidence.

Yoga is a great way to get some exercise and practice mindfulness. Yoga uses breathing and full-body awareness to bring balance and harmony to the mind, body, and soul. Similarly, to essential oils, it is holistic and can be used in conjunction with essential oils. It aims to strengthen the mind, body, and soul through stretching, breathing, and balancing exercises. If you feel like yoga is not for you, Pilates is a similar form of exercise that incorporates core strengthening and breathing as its fundamental teachings.

As you can see, using essential oils as a holistic method of treatment does not only mean putting some oil in a diffuser and hoping for the best. Holistic healing is about being intentional with your existence and the choices you make. However, holistic healing can feel like a lot of pressure. Suddenly, you have to practice mindfulness, meditate, eat healthily, exercise, and still fulfil your other responsibilities? It sounds like a lot, but as you progress in your journey to healing, you will figure out which practices work for you, which ones don't really fit right, and which ones you can adjust to your schedule. The point is that living a healthy and balanced life will supplement the effects of essential oils and other treatments you may be undergoing. If you want your hormones to be balanced, your life has to be balanced.

Chapter 6

A Guide to Essential Oils

This is a guide to essential oils. There are many more essential oils available but the oils identified in this chapter are the most widely accessible. The mentioned oils also offer relief from symptoms of hormonal imbalance. Each of the chosen essential oils will be named by their common and Latin names. This is important information because top-quality essential oil brands include the common and Latin names of the plants. Do not buy essential oils that don't have this information. This guide also provides information on the properties of essential oils, their uses, benefits, best practices, and extra tips and tricks. It offers a comprehensive and accessible encyclopedia-like guide to essential oils that you can use for all of your essential oil needs.

Angelica

Latin name: Angelica Archangelica

Properties: Angelica oil is antispasmodic, which means it can help to relieve spasms and cramps. It has relaxing properties which promote calmness and boost the nervous system. This oil has diuretic and diaphoretic properties which promote urination and sweating. Angelica also helps with digestion and has anti-infection properties.

Uses: Due to its diuretic and diaphoretic properties, it is perfect for detoxifying the body while helping to regulate the metabolism. These properties also promote relief from symptoms caused by gout and arthritis. It reduces levels of anxiety and depression and can help with insomnia. Additionally, it is used to fight off respiratory diseases and coughs. Angelica oil nourishes and revitalizes the skin while soothing irritation.

Best practice: Angelica works best when added to a cream or carrier oil and is applied topically to the skin. Avoid the sun after application as this oil has phototoxic properties and can increase the chances of sunburn.

Tips and tricks: Angelica can help with hiccups. Use the dry evaporation method and take a few deep breaths of the oil for relief from hiccups.

Basil

Latin name: Ocimum Basilicum

Properties: Basil oil can be used as an insect repellent although it is better known for its mood-enhancing properties. It soothes muscle soreness and can keep you alert with its energizing properties. It also helps to regulate digestion and has anti-inflammatory properties.

Uses: Basil can be used to fight respiratory diseases and ease the symptoms of gout. Its mood-enhancing properties mean that it can help with anxiety, depression, mood swings, and feelings of fatigue and tiredness. Basil oil can be used to increase sex drive and improve focus.

Best practice: Basil oil should be added to a carrier oil or cream or inhaled through dry evaporation for optimal effectiveness.

Tips and tricks: Due to its anti-inflammatory properties, basil oil can be used to soothe and cure acne and eczema. You can even add some basil oil to your food when cooking.

Bergamot

Latin name: Citrus Bergamia

Properties: Bergamot has antibacterial and anti-inflammatory properties. It has been found that bergamot oil reduces cholesterol and reduces the amount of fat in the liver. It has analgesic properties, which means that it can alleviate pain.

Uses: Due to its antibacterial and anti-inflammatory properties, it can combat food poisoning, soothe acne, aid in reducing the appearance of sunspots and sun damage, and moisturize the scalp to reduce dandruff. It helps to soothe pain and can be applied to areas with muscle soreness.

Best practice: Bergamot oil can be mixed with a carrier oil or cream and applied to the skin. Adding a few drops to a diffuser is a great way to reap the benefits of bergamot. It also works well in shampoo, conditioner, and body wash.

Tips and tricks: Mixing bergamot and lavender oil can help with sleep and insomnia. It can also help get rid of lice.

Black Pepper

Latin name: Piper Nigrum

Properties: Similarly to angelica oil, black pepper oil has detoxifying qualities as it reduces inflammation in the digestive tract. Black pepper oil also has antiviral and analgesic properties.

Uses: Black pepper oil can be used to reduce and alleviate symptoms of stress and anxiety. Its antiviral properties make it a useful tool to use against viral and respiratory infections. Black pepper oil can be used to provide relief from bloating and constipation due to its anti-inflammatory and detoxifying properties.

Best practice: Black pepper oil should be mixed in a cream or carrier oil and can be applied to the face and chest. The dry evaporation method can be used to relieve symptoms of stress and anxiety.

Tips and tricks: Black pepper oil has been said to reduce nicotine cravings and ease the symptoms of withdrawal when quitting smoking. If you are trying to quit, use the dry evaporation method whenever cravings strike to relieve withdrawal symptoms. Black pepper oil is full of antioxidants and has anti-aging properties. Put a few drops into a face cream for a youthful glow.

Cassia

Latin name: Acacia Farnesiana

Properties: Cassia oil has diuretic and purgative (laxative) properties which make it great for detoxifying. This oil can also bring up mucus which is effective when dealing with illness. Cassia oil boosts the immune system and helps with digestion and blood circulation.

Uses: Cassia oil's detoxifying properties can relieve constipation and diarrhea. It can be used to clear the throat, respiratory tract, and lungs from mucus and can treat a cough. Improved blood circulation means that this oil can be used to alleviate pain, and reduce inflammation and swelling in muscles.

Best practice: Cassia oil can be used in a bath or shower for the full anti-inflammatory effect. It can also be added to a cream or carrier oil to target areas to relieve pain.

Tips and tricks: Cassia oil can reduce menstrual symptoms and regulate periods. It is also a great way to treat arthritis due to its anti-inflammatory properties. It has also been shown to treat diabetes due to its ability to lower blood sugar levels.

Cedarwood

Latin name: Juniperus Virginiana

Properties: Cedarwood has a range of antifungal, antiseptic, anti-inflammatory, and diuretic properties. It also has calming and moisturizing properties.

Uses: Cedarwood can be used for a multitude of different purposes. Its calming properties allow it to treat symptoms of stress and anxiety while also promoting sleep and treating insomnia. It is effective in detoxifying the body due to its diuretic properties. Cedarwood oil can be used to disinfect and treat wounds and scars due to its antiseptic and moisturizing properties. It has also been proven to work in hair regrowth as it stimulates and nourishes hair follicles.

Best practice: Cedarwood is a versatile oil that can be applied to the skin with a cream or carrier oil, diffused, or added to shampoo and body wash.

Tips and tricks: Cedarwood can be found in many colognes and perfumes. It is also known for its insect repellent properties and can serve as a two-in-one perfume and insect repellent.

Cinnamon

Latin name: Cinnamomum Zeylanicum

Properties: Cinnamon oil is known for its heating properties which contribute to the vastness of its uses. It has relaxing properties as well as antifungal and antibacterial properties. It has also been found to be anti-diabetic.

Uses: Due to its heating properties, it is useful for a variety of different uses. These include relieving symptoms of constipation and muscle soreness, and improving digestion. Cinnamon oil can be used to fight infections and reduce the symptoms of stress and anxiety.

Best practice: Cinnamon oil can be massaged into the skin with a cream or carrier oil or added to a diffuser. This oil does not blend with water, so using it in a bath or shower is not advised.

Tips and tricks: Cinnamon oil is effective in preventing cavities and oral thrush due to its antibacterial properties. Place a few drops (diluted in a carrier oil) into the mouth and swish it around for one minute to coat the mouth. Spit the oil out so there is only a thin film left to protect the teeth.

Clove

Latin name: Syzygium Aromaticum

Properties: Like cinnamon oil, clove oil also has heating properties which contribute to its effectiveness. It has analgesic and antimicrobial properties.

Uses: Clove oil is used for a variety of different treatments, including the treatment of headaches, indigestion, respiratory diseases, and other forms of infection due to its analgesic and antibacterial properties. It helps to reduce stress and anxiety and strengthen the immune system.

Best practice: Clove oil is versatile and can be massaged into the skin, diffused, or used as a room and linen spray.

Tips and tricks: Clove oil has been known to relieve toothache due to its analgesic properties. A few drops (diluted in a carrier oil) can be applied to a targeted area. Be sure to avoid the gums as it can cause irritation and burning. A few drops added to a cream and massaged into the skin has also been shown to relieve chronic itching.

Clary Sage

Latin name: Salvia Sclarea

Properties: Clary sage is one of the most versatile and effective essential oils available. It has antidepressant, calming, and relaxing properties, as well as anti-inflammatory and circulation-boosting properties.

Uses: Clary sage oil reduces the effects of stress, anxiety, and depression and also aids in sleep and treating insomnia. It has been known to help with symptoms of menopause and menstrual cramps due to its anti-inflammatory qualities.

Best practice: Clary sage oil can be added to a cream or carrier oil and massaged into targeted areas for pain relief, like the abdomen or temples. It can also be diffused and is one of the few oils that can be safely ingested via smoothies or teas. But remember that ingesting essentials always comes with a risk and only one to two drops should be added.

Tips and tricks: Clary sage is a great oil to use for general household cleaning as it has antibacterial properties and promotes a relaxing aura throughout your home.

Chamomile

Latin name: Anthemis Nobilis

Properties: Chamomile oil has anti-inflammatory properties as well as calming and soothing qualities.

Uses: Chamomile oil is known to reduce symptoms of stress and anxiety while promoting sleep and treating insomnia. It's soothing properties also help to treat acne, rashes, and eczema. While chamomile oil can be used to treat sore muscles, it can also be used to treat back pain and arthritis. It helps to soothe digestive functions and treats flatulence, indigestion, and nausea.

Best practice: Chamomile can be added to a cream or carrier oil and gently massaged into the temples or targeted areas of pain. It can be added to baths and used in a room or linen spray. For pain relief, using a warm compress soaked in water and a few drops of chamomile oil can help to alleviate pain.

Tips and tricks: To help with sleep, make a chamomile linen spray and spritz onto the pillow a few minutes before getting into bed. Drinking chamomile tea while reaping the benefits of the essential oil can be a great way to treat insomnia and anxiety.

Copaiba

Latin name: Copaifera Officinalis

Properties: Copaiba has aphrodisiac qualities as well as anti-inflammatory, analgesic, and antibacterial properties.

Uses: Copaiba can be used to treat various infections, like bladder infections, respiratory infections, and throat infections. It can be used to improve sex drive. Copaiba is also useful in relieving pain and joint soreness and can be used to treat arthritis.

Best practice: Copaiba is best used topically, massaged into the skin or applied with a warm compress.

Tips and tricks: Copaiba oil has protective properties that help to protect the brain from neural disorders and can also protect the liver from liver damage.

Cypress

Latin name: Cupressus Sempervirens

Properties: Cypress oil has cough-suppressing qualities and antibacterial properties.

Uses: There are many uses for cypress oil, including using it to treat hemorrhoids, acne, genital warts, and varicose veins. Cypress oil has also been said to treat cellulite by evening out and moisturizing the skin. The antibacterial properties of cypress oil make it perfect for not only disinfecting wounds but treating scars. The cough-suppressing properties can relieve symptoms of respiratory infections. Cypress oil can also be used to relieve symptoms of stress and anxiety.

Best practice: This oil can be applied topically, diffused, added to a bath, or used in room sprays and body washes.

Tips and tricks: Cypress oil can be used as a body deodorant by rubbing a few diluted drops onto the body to reduce unpleasant odors.

Eucalyptus

Latin name: Eucalyptus Globulus

Properties: Eucalyptus can loosen mucus and has disinfecting properties. This oil also has soothing, analgesic, and anti-inflammatory properties.

Uses: Eucalyptus oil can be used to treat coughs, sinus infections, and chest infections. It is also used to ease back pain and arthritis due to its pain-relieving qualities.

Best practice: Eucalyptus oil is best administered through steam inhalation by placing your head over a bowl of warm water and eucalyptus oil or by adding a few drops to a bath. You can also add a few drops of eucalyptus oil to a cream or carrier oil and apply it on the chest and under the nose.

Tips and tricks: Eucalyptus oil can be used in a sauna or steam room to clear the chest and nasal cavities. It can also help to treat asthma and, if you like to go camping, it can be used as a tick repellent. Also, if you struggle with bad breath, eucalyptus oil can be found in quite a few mouthwashes. It will disinfect your mouth and leave it feeling fresh.

Fennel

Latin name: Foeniculum Vulgare

Properties: Fennel contains antioxidants and has soothing properties. Like most essential oils, it has anti-inflammatory and antibacterial properties

Uses: Fennel oil can be used to moisturize the skin and treat rashes, acne, and eczema. It can also be used to nourish and heal the hair. Fennel helps with digestion and can alleviate the symptoms of irritable bowel syndrome.

Best practice: Fennel oil can be rubbed onto the bottom of the feet to help with digestion. It can also be diffused or applied topically to soothe targeted areas of the body and for a general calming effect.

Tips and tricks: Fennel oil can be used to control weight gain as it has appetite-suppressing qualities. Add a few drops to toothpaste to curb appetite. Fennel oil is also believed to provide protection against the sun and can be applied to the skin. However, when using fennel oil with a carrier oil, the effect may be offset by the carrier oil which will most likely cause sunburn instead of preventing it. Instead, add a few drops of fennel oil to a cream that already contains SPF (Sun Protection Factor).

Frankincense

Latin name: Boswellia

Properties: Frankincense has relaxing and calming properties. It reduces inflammation and has analgesic properties.

Uses: The relaxing properties of frankincense oil can alleviate headaches and treat symptoms of stress and anxiety. This oil aids in sleep and treats insomnia. It can also be used to treat arthritis by reducing pain and increasing the mobility of the joints.

Best practice: Frankincense oil can be taken in tablet form but can also be added to creams and carrier oils to be massaged onto the skin.

Tips and tricks: Daily doses of frankincense oil can help to alleviate symptoms of asthma and reduce the frequency and intensity of asthma attacks.

Geranium

Latin name: Pelargonium Graveolens

Properties: Geranium oil has anti-aging and antioxidant qualities, along with anti-inflammatory, analgesic, calming, and antibacterial properties.

Uses: It is a useful ingredient in creams and beauty products due to its anti-aging and antioxidant properties. It helps to nourish, revitalize, and plump the skin. It's antibacterial properties also make it safe to use on the skin to treat acne and pimples. Geranium oil has also been shown to reduce anxiety, alleviate pain, and ease swelling.

Best practice: Geranium oil can be applied to the skin with a cream of carrier oil or diffused.

Tips and tricks: Not only can it be used to moisturize the skin but it can be used as a face cleanser as it removes dead skin cells and inhibits the growth of bacteria. Add a few drops to your face wash and use once a day.

Grapefruit

Latin name: Citrus Racemosa

Properties: Grapefruit oil has mood-enhancing, soothing, and antibacterial properties. This oil can also lower blood pressure and improve circulation.

Uses: Grapefruit oil is a natural mood enhancer and, unlike most of the oils explored in this guide, won't put you to sleep. This oil, while it has relaxing and de-stressing properties, also has the ability to wake you up and give you a rush of energy.

Best practice: Grapefruit oil is best used by dry evaporation and diffusion but can be mixed into a cream or carrier oil and massaged onto the skin.

Tips and tricks: Grapefruit oil can be used to control weight gain as it has appetite-suppressing properties. Use the dry evaporation method whenever you feel a craving coming on to prevent overeating. It can also be used to treat the symptoms of a hangover and jet lag.

Ginger

Latin name: Zingiber Officinale

Properties: Ginger has natural heating properties which provide relief from inflammation. It has antibacterial, growth-stimulating, and antioxidant properties.

Uses: Ginger oil is effective in alleviating nausea. It is also a useful treatment for colds and flu. Ginger oil balances the digestive system and ensures gut health. It can also be used to stimulate hair growth and soothe redness and swelling of the face.

Best practice: Ginger oil is a versatile essential oil and can be topically applied, diffused, added to linen and room sprays, added to baths and showers, and inhaled with steam.

Tips and tricks: Ginger oil has also been found to work as an aphrodisiac and improve sex drive. Add a few drops of ginger oil to a diffuser for optimal effect.

Hyssop

Latin name: Hyssopus Officinalis

Properties: Hyssop has anti-inflammatory, antibacterial, and antioxidant properties. It can also loosen mucus and fight infection.

Uses: Hyssop oil can be used to alleviate the symptoms and effects of respiratory infections and coughs. It can be used to treat asthma. Hyssop oil can strengthen the response to external toxins and slows down the aging process. It can also be used to alleviate pain.

Best practice: Hyssop can be diffused, applied topically, added to a warm compress, steamed, or added to a bath.

Tips and tricks: Hyssop oil should not be ingested. It should also not be taken during pregnancy as it may result in miscarriage.

Jasmine

Latin name: Jasminum Grandiflorum

Properties: Jasmine oil has many beneficial qualities, including antiseptic, antidepressant, soothing, aphrodisiac, and antispasmodic properties.

Uses: Jasmine oil can be used to disinfect and treat wounds and infection. It can also be used to increase sex drive and enhance mood. It has calming properties, which means that it can help with sleep and treat insomnia. Jasmine's antispasmodic properties also prevents muscle spasms and soothes muscle soreness.

Best practice: Jasmine oil can be applied topically, diffused, inhaled through steam, added to a warm bath, or added to linen and room sprays.

Tips and tricks: Jasmine oil can help to calm the nerves. Use the dry evaporation method and take a few deep breaths before you have to give a big presentation, or if you are on the verge of a panic attack.

Juniper

Latin name: Juniperus Communis

Properties: Juniper oil has antioxidant, anti-inflammatory, and antibacterial properties. It also has analgesic qualities.

Uses: Juniper oil can be used to purify the air. This is especially useful if you live in the city or a generally polluted area. Juniper oil can relieve pain and numb targeted areas and is a great skin cleanser due to its anti-inflammatory properties.

Best practice: Juniper oil can be inhaled with steam to help treat bronchitis. It can also be added to face wash and face toners to plumb, revitalize, and clean skin.

Tips and tricks: Juniper oil can be used to treat ringworm. Add a few drops of diluted oil to a cotton ball and apply to the affected area.

Lavender

Latin name: Lavandula Angustifolia

Properties: Lavender oil has a wide array of benefits. It has calming, soothing, antidepressant, and anti-anxiety properties. It also has antiseptic, antibacterial, and anti-inflammatory qualities.

Uses: Lavender oil can be used to alleviate symptoms of stress, anxiety, and depression. It is used in a wide variety of soaps and cleansers due to its calming aroma. It's antibacterial and antiseptic properties are useful in disinfecting and treating wounds and scars. Lavender oil also helps with sleep and treats insomnia.

Best practice: Lavender oil can be added to a cream or carrier oil and massaged onto the skin. It can be diffused, inhaled through steam, added to shampoo and body wash, added to baths and showers, and added to linen and room sprays. It can also be inhaled through the dry evaporation method.

Tips and tricks: Lavender oil can ease muscle soreness and increase mobility in joints. This is why it is used during massages and other therapeutic treatments. Add a few drops to a carrier oil and massage it into your temples, neck, and shoulders to relieve stress and tension.

Lemon

Latin name: Citrus Limonum

Properties: Lemon has antibacterial properties, which is why it can be found in many household cleaning products. It also has calming and soothing properties.

Uses: Lemon oil can be used to fight symptoms of colds and flu due to its antibacterial properties. It is also used to disinfect wounds and treat acne. It has been known to help with anxiety and depression and can leave you feeling energized. Lemon oil has also been shown to improve skin by reducing inflammation and removing bacteria.

Best practice: Lemon oil is best used by applying it topically with a cream or carrier oil to the skin or diffusing it into a well-ventilated space.

Tips and tricks: Lemon oil can be used to treat morning sickness. Place a few drops in a diffuser at night to wake up with a lemon-scented room and no morning sickness. It is best to avoid the sun after application of lemon oil.

Lemongrass

Latin name: Cymbopogon

Properties: Lemongrass has anti-inflammatory, antiseptic, analgesic, and antifungal properties.

Uses: Lemongrass oil can be used to clean wounds, treat respiratory infections, and treat fungal infections, like athlete's foot. It can be used to reduce blood sugar levels and improve cardiovascular function. It helps to refresh skin with its antioxidants. Lemongrass oil can also be used to treat headaches, muscle pain, and relieve symptoms of stress and anxiety.

Best practice: Lemongrass oil can be applied to the skin with a cream or carrier oil, added to shampoo or body wash, and inhaled through dry evaporation.

Tips and tricks: A few drops of lemongrass oil can be added to mouthwash to stop gingivitis and fungal infections.

Mandarin

Latin name: Citrus Reticulata

Properties: Manadin oil is a gentle essential oil with antioxidants. It has anti-inflammatory properties and enhances mood.

Uses: Mandarin oil is used to minimize and treat scarring and stretch marks. It is also said to uplift the mood with its fresh and bright aroma. It can soothe skin irritation and helps to nourish the skin.

Best practice: Mandarin oil is best applied to the skin with a cream or carrier oil or diffused into a room.

Tips and tricks: Add a few drops to a diffuser in your office so that you can maintain a bright and cheery aura even if the work is boring and stressful.

Marigold

Latin name: Calendula Officinalis

Properties: Marigold oil (also commonly referred to as calendula oil) has incredible healing powers. It has antibacterial, antifungal, antiseptic, and antimicrobial properties. It also has soothing and anti-inflammatory properties.

Uses: Marigold oil can be used to treat acne, rashes, diaper rashes, skin irritation, and eczema. It can be used to disinfect and treat wounds and promotes youthful skin.

Best practice: Marigold oil is best applied to the skin with a cream or carrier oil.

Tips and tricks: Marigold oil can be used as a sunscreen when added to cream. However, for safety reasons, add a few drops into a cream that already has proven SPF properties.

Melissa

Latin name: Melissa Officinalis

Properties: Melissa oil (also commonly referred to as lemon balm) can be used to treat a wide array of illnesses and infections due to its antibacterial and soothing properties.

Uses: Melissa oil can be used to treat bronchitis and relieve the symptoms of colds and flu. This oil can also be applied to cold sores and eczema. It helps to soothe and treat the symptoms of stress and anxiety, and can also have an energizing effect on the body and mind.

Best practice: Melissa oil is best used when applied to the skin with a cream or carrier oil, diffused, or inhaled using the dry evaporation method.

Tips and tricks: Melissa oil helps with allergies and can be added to a diffuser or inhaled through the dry evaporation method to make sure you get through allergy season unscathed.

Myrrh

Latin name: Commiphora Myrrha

Properties: Myrrh oil has anti-inflammatory and antibacterial properties.

Uses: Myrrh oil can be used to clean and disinfect wounds, and also helps to reduce swelling and pain. It can be used to soothe headaches and muscle pain. Myrrh oil can also be used to treat athlete's foot and ringworm.

Best practice: Myrrh oil can be applied to the skin with a cream or carrier oil and added to shampoo or shower gel. It can also be inhaled with a diffuser and applied to the mouth to treat cold sores but should not be ingested.

Tips and tricks: Myrrh can be rubbed onto walls and cupboards where mold occurs to prevent the growth of mildew and other fungus.

Oregano

Latin name: Origanum Vulgare

Properties: Oregano isn't just great in pasta. This generous oil has antimicrobial, antioxidant, and anti-inflammatory properties.

Uses: Oregano oil can be used to treat urinary tract infections as well as other bacterial and fungal infections including yeast infections, respiratory infections, and athlete's foot. It reduces bloating and can be an effective tool in fighting parasites in the gut. Oregano oil has also been shown to reduce cholesterol and aid in weight loss.

Best practice: Oregano oil can be ingested in tablet form but it can also be applied to the skin with a cream or carrier oil.

Tips and tricks: Oregano has been shown to combat bacteria that is resistant to antibiotics and can be effective as an antibiotic itself. Oregano oil can also be used to treat a cold. Add a few drops to hot water and steam for two to three minutes.

Orange

Latin name: Citrus Sinensis

Properties: Orange oil has energizing properties, as well as antioxidant, anti-inflammatory, and antibacterial properties.

Uses: Due to its energizing properties, orange oil can be used to maintain focus, increase performance and relieve symptoms of anxiety and depression. It can also be used to treat acne and revitalize skin. Due to its anti-inflammatory properties, orange oil can reduce pain, swelling, and treat digestive issues.

Best practice: Avoid using this oil before bedtime as it will increase alertness instead of inducing sleep. Orange oil can be applied to the skin with a cream or carrier oil or diffused into a room or place of work to keep you focused and energized.

Tips and tricks: Orange oil can help with physical performance. Use the dry evaporation method and take a few deep breaths before hitting the gym or going for a hike. It's the perfect remedy after a long work week or sleepless night.

Patchouli

Latin name: Pogostemon Cablin

Properties: Patchouli oil has anti-inflammatory, analgesic, and antibacterial properties.

Uses: Patchouli oil is a good tool to use for skincare. It smoothes skin, evens complexion, and has hydrating properties. It also helps with acne and dry skin. It can be used to relieve depression and ease feelings of stress and anxiety. It can also be used for weight loss as it has appetite-suppressing properties.

Best practice: Patchouli oil can be applied to the skin with a cream or carrier oil. It can also be diffused or inhaled through steam or dry evaporation methods.

Tips and tricks: Patchouli oil has been shown to increase collagen which decreases wrinkle formation.

Add a few drops to your night cream to wake up to a fresh, plump, and wrinkle-free face.

Peppermint

Latin name: Mentha Piperita

Properties: Peppermint oil is a great essential oil to have on hand at all times. It has analgesic properties and can help with digestion. It also has energizing properties.

Uses: Peppermint oil's energizing properties promote hair growth and bright skin. It also improves focus and can be used to enhance mood and balance mood swings. This oil can alleviate pain caused by irritable bowel syndrome or general digestion issues and also helps to ease feelings of nausea. Peppermint oil has antifungal and antibacterial properties and can be used to treat various yeast and bacterial infections.

Best practice: Peppermint oil can be added to a cream or carrier oil and applied to the skin. It can also be diffused or inhaled through the dry evaporation method.

Tips and tricks: Add peppermint oil to a room spray at work to maintain focus and keep the energy going.

Rose

Latin name: Rosa Damascena

Properties: Rose oil is great for the skin as it has nourishing, hydrating, anti-aging, and anti-inflammatory properties.

Uses: Rose oil is present in many skincare products and can be used to clear acne, revitalize and hydrate skin, and even out complexion by removing and soothing scars, wrinkles, and stretch marks. It can also be used to treat eczema. Rose oil is an aphrodisiac and can be used to boost the sex drive. It also protects against infection and bacteria and alleviates pain. Rose oil also helps ease the symptoms of stress, anxiety, and depression.

Best practice: Rose oil can be added to a cream or carrier oil and applied to the skin. It can be added to linen and room sprays, diffused, or added to a bath.

Tips and tricks: Apply a few drops to a warm compress to help alleviate a headache or any kind of inflammation and muscle soreness.

Rosemary

Latin name: Rosmarinus Officinalis

Properties: Rosemary oil has anti-inflammatory, energizing, and cognitive enhancing properties. It is also antibacterial and has antioxidant properties.

Uses: Rosemary oil has been known to stimulate hair growth. It can also be used to maintain focus, improve alertness, and improve memory. Rosemary oil helps with stress and anxiety and can also relieve pain. It regulates blood circulation and can alleviate joint soreness and stiffness.

Best practice: Rosemary oil can be mixed with a cream or carrier oil and applied topically. It can also be diffused, or inhaled through the steam inhalation or dry evaporation methods.

Tips and tricks: Rosemary oil can help with baldness. Add a few drops to a cream or carrier oil of your choice and massage it into the scalp for several minutes a day.

Sage

Latin name: Salvia Officinalis

Properties: Sage oil has antibacterial, cleansing, and anti-inflammatory properties. It is more robust than clary sage oil which is gentler and sweeter. Sage oil has decongestant, anesthetic, antispasmodic, and analgesic properties.

Uses: Sage oil can be used to reduce swelling and pain as well as to reduce the frequency and intensity of muscle spasms. It also helps to disinfect and heal wounds. Due to its decongestant properties, sage oil can be used to alleviate the symptoms of nasal congestion, respiratory infections, and throat infections.

Best practice: Sage oil is best added to a cream or carrier oil and applied to the affected areas. It can be added to a warm compress or inhaled through steam inhalation.

Tips and tricks: Sage oil can be used as a face cleanser to remove excess sebum and dirt from the face. Add a few drops to your face wash or face cleanser for cleaner, brighter skin.

Sandalwood

Latin name: Santalum Spicatum

Properties: Sandalwood has antiseptic, antibacterial, anti-inflammatory, and antifungal properties. It also has purifying and soothing properties.

Uses: Sandalwood can be used to relieve stress and anxiety and promote sleep. It also has balancing and detoxifying properties which treat indigestion, liver issues, and urinary tract infections. It can be used to lower blood pressure and alleviate fatigue. Sandalwood can disinfect and treat wounds and infections.

Best practice: Sandalwood can be added to a cream or carrier oil and applied topically. It can also be diffused, added to a bath, added to a room or linen spray, and inhaled using the steam inhalation or dry evaporation methods.

Tips and tricks: Sandalwood oil controls the amount of oil on the face and can be used on oily skin and also to treat acne. Add a few drops to a face cream for balanced skin.

Spearmint

Latin name: Mentha Spicata

Properties: Spearmint oil has anti-inflammatory and analgesic properties. It is considered to be gentler than peppermint oil. It has diuretic, antispasmodic, and relaxing properties.

Uses: Spearmint oil can be useful in treating digestive issues, like irritable bowel syndrome and general digestion. It also has detoxifying properties and can reduce stress and anxiety. It can be used to enhance focus and concentration. Because it is gentler than peppermint oil, it can be used to reduce redness, even out complexion, and hydrate the skin on the face.

Best practice: Spearmint oil works best when added to a cream or carrier oil and applied to the skin. It can also be diffused, added to a bath, added to a room spray, or inhaled through the dry evaporation method.

Tips and tricks: Spearmint oil can be added to face cleansers and face wash to promote skin elasticity and tighten pores.

Tea Tree

Latin name: Melaleuca Alternifolia

Properties: Tea tree oil is one of those super oils that just seems to help with everything. It has antiseptic, antibacterial, and antifungal properties.

Uses: Tea tree oil can be used to disinfect and clean wounds and speeds up the healing process. It has been known to treat acne and nail fungus. It can be used as a natural hand sanitizer. Tea tree oil has drying properties and can therefore be used to treat oily and itchy skin. It helps to reduce inflammation which makes it a great cure for acne and eczema and also helps with psoriasis.

Best practice: Tea tree oil is best diluted in a cream or carrier oil and applied directly to the skin and affected areas.

Tips and tricks: Tea tree oil can be used as a natural deodorant. Add a few drops to a carrier oil and place under the arms, behind the ears, and on the wrists.

Thyme

Latin name: Thymus Vulgaris

Properties: Thyme has antimicrobial, antifungal, and antibacterial properties.

Uses: Thyme oil is used in a variety of mouthwashes. It inhibits the growth of acne, producing bacteria and can also promote hair growth.

Best practice: Thyme oil can be used as a mouthwash (just remember not to ingest it). It can also be added to a cream or carrier oil and applied to the skin.

Tips and tricks: Thyme oil can be added to hot water and breathed in through steam inhalation to help with coughing and respiratory infections.

Wintergreen

Latin name: Gaultheria Procumbens

Properties: Wintergreen oil has anti-inflammatory and analgesic properties.

Uses: Wintergreen oil can increase the amount of stomach acid produced by the pancreas, aiding in digestion. It can also alleviate pain from sore muscles and joints. It helps to prevent tooth decay by cleaning plaque and preventing gingivitis.

Best practice: Add to a cream or carrier oil and apply to the affected areas of the skin.

Tips and tricks: Add a few drops to a warm compress and place it on the lower back or head to relieve back pain and headaches.

Ylang-Ylang

Latin name: Cananga Odorata

Properties: Ylang-ylang oil has mood-enhancing, antibacterial, and aphrodisiac properties.

Uses: Ylang-ylang oil can be used to treat anxiety and depression and relieve symptoms of stress. It also helps to lower heart rate and blood pressure. It has been shown to treat gout.

Best practice: Ylang-ylang oil can be added to a cream or carrier oil and applied to the skin or diffused. It can also be added to a linen spray to help with sleep.

Tips and tricks: Add a few drops of ylang-ylang oil to a carrier oil and apply to skin and scalp to prevent dryness, rehydrate the skin, and prevent dandruff.

Part 3:

A Guide to Hormonal Imbalance and Treating Symptoms with Essential Oils

Chapter 7

Physiological Symptoms of Hormonal Imbalance

Understanding the properties and uses of essential oils is crucial to the next step of the process. It is also useful to have a guide on hand for when you are experiencing a little bit of inflammation or a touch of skin discoloration. Having an encyclopedia-like reference point is like having a roadmap of essential oils. However, this knowledge can be somewhat redundant if you don't know how, when, and why to use the oils. In this chapter, and the two after this, you will find a comprehensive guide to hormonal imbalance symptoms and how essential oils can help treat them. The chapters are divided into physiological, mental, and other symptoms of hormonal imbalance to provide a thorough list of possible symptoms that can be caused by hormonal imbalance. If the symptoms you experience are not included on this list, consult a doctor and use the essential oil guide to decide on the best possible course of action for your symptoms.

Acne

Definition: Acne can have varying degrees of severity. It is a skin condition that causes swelling, scarring, oily skin, and red bumps filled with pus on the face, back, and neck areas. Acne can be caused by hormonal imbalances catalyzed by puberty, pregnancy, and even menopause.

Symptoms: The symptoms of acne include red bumps on the body that are filled with pus. Often, these are painful.

Treatment: Tea tree oil can be effective in treating acne because it has anti-inflammatory, antibacterial, and drying properties which help to reduce inflammation, swelling, and redness. Basil, bergamot, and chamomile oil also help to soothe acne.

Best practice: Add a few drops to a cream or carrier oil and apply to the face daily. A few drops can also be added to a bowl of hot water to steam the face. This hydrates and cleans the face.

Tips and tricks: Add a few drops of juniper oil to your face wash and cleanse your face before applying a tea tree oil enriched cream. It is best to add the essential oil to a cream instead of a carrier oil to reduce the amount of oil on the face, which can often cause pimples.

Adrenal Fatigue

Definition: Adrenal fatigue is a condition that occurs when the adrenal glands are not functioning properly. The adrenal gland controls the levels of cortisol in the body. In periods of extreme or chronic stress, the adrenal gland can become fatigued and stops functioning as it should. This leads to poor stress responses as the levels of cortisol in the body are no longer regulated appropriately. Think of it as a marathon. You start the race all enthusiastic and energetic, and as you go on, you start to get slower, more tired, and your legs start to drag as you fling your body to the finish line only to find that you have fallen a few feet short. Similarly, the adrenal gland starts enthusiastically and releases cortisol because the body is stressed and the adrenal gland has got it all under control. But the stress doesn't stop and the adrenal gland has to keep up with the level of stress but it's struggling as it drags its cortisol producing abilities to the finish line and flings itself a few feet short. The adrenal gland is tired and needs a breather before it can continue producing cortisol as it should.

Symptoms: Adrenal fatigue can lead to tiredness, mood swings, and brain fog. Cortisol also helps to regulate the body's blood pressure and adrenal fatigue may lead to higher or lower levels of blood pressure.

Treatment: Orange, peppermint, lemon, and grapefruit oil can help to keep you energized and reduce brain fog. Cedarwood and chamomile oil can be used to increase relaxation and promote calm in times of high stress. Ylang-ylang oil can be used to stabilize mood swings.

Best practice: Diffuse a few drops of these oils into your room or workplace or take a few deep breaths, using the dry evaporation method for an instant pick-me-up.

Tips and tricks: Adrenal fatigue is your body's way of telling you to slow down. So draw a bubble bath, add a few drops of lavender oil, spray some linen spray infused with jasmine oil on your bedsheets and get ready for an evening of relaxation. The deadline can wait, right now your adrenal gland needs some love.

Amenorrhea

Definition: This is the absence of a period. It can be due to pregnancy, stress, or menopause. However, it is not the same as having irregular periods. A woman is diagnosed with amenorrhea once they have missed three consecutive periods.

Symptoms: The symptoms are varying and can result in acne, excessive hair growth or hair loss, headaches, and nipple discharge. Amenorrhea may be caused by certain medications, contraceptives, and diet. For example, people suffering from anorexia often experience amenorrhea.

Treatment: Clary sage oil can be used to balance female hormones, primarily estrogen and progesterone. This is a prime example of how holistic healing and taking care of the mental, physical, and spiritual elements can help cure certain conditions. Often, amenorrhea can be cured by maintaining a balanced diet, eating regularly, not exercising too much, and finding medications that don't cause amenorrhea. Sandalwood oil can be used to regulate androgen levels in the body and help to reduce the effects of hair loss and excess hair growth, and tea tree oil can be used to treat acne.

Best practice: To relieve the symptoms of amenorrhea, add a few drops of clary sage oil to a warm compress and place it on the abdominal area. Sandalwood oil can be added to a bath to regulate androgen levels.

Tips and tricks: When using essential oils to treat amenorrhea, make sure you are eating a healthy and balanced diet.

Androgen Deficiency

Definition: Androgen deficiency refers to reduced levels of male hormones, mainly testosterone. This can occur in males and females.

Symptoms: The symptoms of androgen deficiency include low sex drive, decreased muscle mass, fatigue, erectile dysfunction, depression, and mood swings.

Treatment: Many different symptoms are caused by androgen deficiency and require specific treatment to help ease these symptoms. For fatigue, orange and grapefruit oil can re-energize you. Jasmine, copaiba, ginger, rose, and ylang-ylang oil all have aphrodisiac properties and can increase the sex drive. Cassia, clary sage, rosemary, and grapefruit oil aid in increasing circulation, a property that can help to manage erectile dysfunction. Lavender oil and ylang-ylang oil can be used to relieve depression and manage mood swings.

Best practice: Grapefruit and ylang-ylang are the common denominators in the treatment suggestions and can therefore be diffused into a room or you can take a few deep breaths using the dry evaporation method.

Tips and tricks: Minimizing stress is one of the best ways to help with androgen deficiency. While other oils can provide relief from symptoms, managing levels of stress and anxiety can yield quicker results. So, make sure to take a few moments a day to practice mindfulness and relax.

Arthritis

Definition: Arthritis refers to the inflammation of joints which causes stiffness and pain. There are several different forms of arthritis but the most common are rheumatoid arthritis and osteoarthritis. The former is an autoimmune disease. Essentially, the body attacks its own tissue, thus causing inflammation, swelling, and pain in the joints. The latter is due to the overuse of joints and can get worse with age.

Symptoms: Symptoms caused by arthritis may include, but are not limited to, swelling, inflammation, pain, fatigue, and stiffness.

Treatment: Angelica, cassia, copaiba, chamomile, eucalyptus, and frankincense oil are the most effective in treating and relieving the symptoms of arthritis. They have anti-inflammatory properties which help to ease swelling and pain in the joints. Copaiba, eucalyptus, and frankincense oil have analgesic properties to help ease the pain caused by arthritis.

Best practice: The best way to use these oils to treat symptoms of arthritis is by adding a few drops to a warm compress or taking a warm bath. It is also possible to add a few drops to a cream or carrier oil and apply directly to the affected joints for relief.

Tips and tricks: Arthritis can also be treated by making a *cocktail* of essential oils. Add a few drops of eucalyptus, lavender, chamomile, frankincense, and copaiba oil to a cream or carrier oil and apply to affected areas. Remember to maintain an acceptable essential oil to carrier oil ratio.

Bloating

Definition: Bloating is the presence of excess gas in the stomach. Besides making you feel uncomfortable, it can also be painful. Having high levels of estrogen in the body can lead to bloating but it is caused by eating too much food too quickly, or drinking carbonated drinks. Bloating can also be caused by constipation.

Symptoms: Bloating causes the stomach to expand and may increase flatulence and burping. It can also result in abdominal pain due to trapped gas.

Treatment: Ginger and peppermint oil are the go-to oils when treating digestive and abdominal issues. Chamomile can also help to soothe the stomach and intestines so that you can wait for the gas to pass painlessly.

Best practice: These oils are best applied with a warm compress to the abdominal area. This can help relieve pain and speed up the digestion process.

Tips and tricks: If you struggle with bloating, try exercising for a few minutes a day or going for a walk to speed up your metabolism. This will get your digestive system going and can ease bloating faster.

Blurred Vision

Definition: Blurred vision refers to a decrease in the functioning of the eye. This could be as a result of dizziness or due to certain hormonal changes, like menopause. Increased levels of estrogen and progesterone in the body can cause the cornea of the eye (the part of the eye that controls the light that enters the eye) to become elastic which results in blurred vision.

Symptoms: Blurred vision caused by hormonal imbalance is not constant but fluctuating. It can lead to headaches, strained and pained eyes, light sensitivity, and dryness in the eye.

Treatment: Sandalwood oil can help to bring balance back to the hormone secreted by the ovaries, mainly estrogen and progesterone. Lavender oil can be used to treat headaches and rose oil has analgesic properties to help with pain.

Best practice: Essential oils should not be applied to the eyes, which may make blurred vision difficult to treat. This is why it is crucial to treat the cause (which is hormonal imbalance) rather than the effect (which is blurred vision, in this case). Add a few drops of lavender oil to a cream or carrier oil and massage into the temples for headache relief. Add a few drops of sandalwood oil to a bath or diffuser or gently massage cream into the abdominal area and temples.

Tips and tricks: If your eyes are feeling fatigued, take a few deep breaths of orange oil to refocus them, and if they are feeling strained, try a more calming oil, like rose or chamomile, to relax them.

Bone Density

Definition: Bone density refers to the health, strength, and mineral ratio of the bones in the body. Having good bone density means that the bones have enough minerals to keep the body upright, prevent fractures, and protect organs. Low bone density can lead to osteoporosis and bone fractures. Think of it as one of those life-size skeletons that doctors sometimes have in their offices. The skeleton has no bone density and, therefore, if the wires holding it up were removed, it would collapse. Similarly, while humans do have muscles and other things to hold them upright, without any bone density, without any structural integrity, they wouldn't be able to stand. Bone density can be affected by imbalanced estrogen and testosterone levels and imbalances within the pituitary, parathyroid, and thyroid glands.

Symptoms: A condition caused by low bone density is osteoporosis which leads to back pain, bad posture, weak bones, and trouble standing.

Treatment: Sandalwood oil helps to balance estrogen levels while cedarwood helps to balance testosterone levels. Thyme and rosemary oil have recently been studied and are said to prevent osteoporosis and strengthen bones (Elbanhnasawy, 2019). Although the study was performed on rats, the results were nonetheless promising. Lemongrass oil can also be used to balance the thyroid gland.

Best practice: Add a few drops of essential oils to a cream or carrier oil and massage the body. Warm compresses also help but the chances are that bone density is experienced throughout the body and not in targeted areas. This means that a bath can help to balance hormones.

Tips and tricks: Remember to eat your vegetables! They will, in conjunction with essential oils, give your bones the minerals required to get stronger.

Candida

Definition: Candida is a type of fungus that is most commonly used to identify oral and vaginal thrush. It causes a white, cotton-like mucus to form and can often cause an odor. Candida is also contagious which is why it is necessary to get it treated as soon as possible.

Symptoms: Candida can result in feelings of fatigue, skin irritation, and infections.

Treatment: Lemongrass and thyme oil can be used for oral thrush as they are present in many types of mouthwashes and have antifungal properties which can stifle the growth of candida. Tea tree oil can be used to disinfect the affected areas.

Best practice: For vaginal thrush, take a warm bath with a few drops of tea tree oil and a few tablespoons of baking soda. This will help to neutralize the fungus and disinfect the area. For oral thrush, add a few drops of thyme or lemongrass oil to toothpaste or on a toothbrush, brush teeth gently for a few minutes every day for several days until symptoms subside.

Tips and tricks: Do not apply or insert undiluted or diluted essential oils into the vaginal cavity. This can cause irritation, swelling, and burning.

Cushing's Disease

Definition: Cushing's disease is caused by prolonged exposure to high levels of cortisol in the body. It stems from an imbalance in the adrenal gland which causes it to overproduce cortisol.

Symptoms: Symptoms may include, but are not limited to, sweating, fatigue, increased appetite, high blood pressure, acne, hair loss, insomnia, stretch marks, and depression. Signs of Cushing's disease include a rounder or swollen face and a fatty pocket of tissue at the base of the neck.

Treatment: Due to the high levels of cortisol in the body, relaxation is crucial. Lavender, sandalwood, jasmine, and rose oil can lower levels of cortisol and give the adrenal glands a break. To reduce swelling in the face, tea tree oil and frankincense oil can reduce inflammation and tea tree oil can also help to eliminate stretch marks.

Best practice: Add lavender, rose, jasmine, and sandalwood oil to a diffuser or a bath for ultimate relaxation. Add a few drops to a cream or carrier oil and rub into the temples, head, neck, shoulders, and lower back (close to your kidneys) for relaxation. Tea tree oil can be added to a cream or carrier oil to help with inflammation, swelling, and stretch marks.

Tips and tricks: These oils can also be mixed and diffused for an extra dose of essential oil therapy.

Diabetes

Definition: There are several kinds of diabetes. Generally, diabetes deals with the level of sugar in the body. Being prediabetic means that blood sugar levels are high but can be reversed. Type 1 diabetes is when the pancreas fails to produce enough, or any, insulin to regulate blood sugar levels in the body. Type 2 diabetes refers to how the body handles blood sugar in the body. Diabetes is mainly caused by poor lifestyle choices like an unhealthy diet but can also be caused by genes. Diabetes is the result of an imbalance of the insulin hormone produced by the pancreas.

Symptoms: Prediabetes often does not present symptoms and the diagnosis is made when blood sugar levels are checked. Type 1 and 2 diabetes can cause fatigue, blurred vision, nausea, weight loss, and abnormal urination.

Treatment: Cassia oil has been known to boost the immune system and regulate sugar levels in the body.

Best practice: Add a few drops of cassia oil to a cream or carrier oil and apply to the abdominal area. Adding a few drops to a diffuser or bath can also help to boost the immune system and regulate sugar levels.

Tips and tricks: If you have a sweet tooth but also have diabetes, then you might struggle to satisfy your sweet cravings. Adding a few drops of cinnamon oil to a diffuser can give you a hit of sweetness without putting you at risk.

Digestive Issues

Definition: Digestive issues also deal with a wide variety of conditions that will also be explored individually. This section will explain general discomfort and pain felt in the stomach and intestines, and how to bring balance back to your gut. Having an imbalanced gut can reduce the effectiveness of the digestive system in absorbing nutrients, storing fat, and digesting food.

Symptoms: Symptoms may include pain and discomfort in the abdominal area, irregular bowel movements, tiredness, and fluctuating weight.

Treatment: For good gut health, peppermint and spearmint are the perfect oils to reset the digestive system and bring balance back to the body.

Best practice: Add a few drops of essential oil to a cream or carrier oil and gently rub into the abdominal area for relief from digestive pain. A warm compress or bath can also be effective in reducing symptoms. Add a few drops to a diffuser or inhale with the dry evaporation method for gut balance.

Tips and tricks: Ginger and spearmint oil both have properties that aid with digestion and can therefore be mixed to form a holistic treatment for an imbalanced gut. The spearmint oil is gentle and can help with irritable bowel syndrome, as well as general digestion, while ginger oil protects the stomach.

Excessive Sweating

Definition: Excessive sweating refers to sweating that does not occur due to exercise or heat and occurs more frequently and in greater quantity. Excessive sweating is often brought about by hyper- and hypothyroidism as a result of a hormonal imbalance in the thyroid gland.

Symptoms: Symptoms include profuse sweating from the underarms, face, and other parts of the body.

Treatment: Rose geranium and frankincense oil can be used to manage the symptoms of hormonal imbalance in the thyroid gland. Tea tree oil can also reduce the amount of sweating due to its drying properties.

Best practice: Add a few drops of essential oil to a cream or carrier oil and apply to the affected areas. If sweating occurs mostly under the arms, apply the cream or oil to the area. Add a few drops of oil to a bath so that the body and sweat glands can absorb the essential oils and reduce the amount of sweating.

Tips and tricks: Tea tree oil also acts as a natural deodorant so not only can it help you to sweat less but it can also make you smell nice.

Eczema

Definition: Eczema is an inflammation of the skin that appears as a rash on the body.

Symptoms: Eczema is often itchy and results in dry and rough skin. It can cause swelling, discoloration and increases the sensitivity of the skin.

Treatment: Basil, chamomile, fennel, melissa, marigold, and rose oil are all effective in treating the symptoms of eczema. They hydrate the skin, which eases symptoms of itching. These oils are also anti-inflammatory which means they can reduce swelling, redness, and general pain associated with inflammation.

Best practice: Essential oils should be diluted in a cream or carrier oil and applied directly to the affected areas. If eczema has spread to several areas on the body then a warm bath with a few drops of oil will help to relieve some of the symptoms.

Tips and tricks: Add a few drops of essential oil to a humidifier. The water vapor will help hydrate the skin while the essential oil works its magic.

Headaches

Definition: Headaches refer to the pain experienced in parts of the head. This can be due to eye strain, stress, noise levels, low blood sugar levels, and low levels of estrogen.

Symptoms: The symptoms of a headache include a dull or sharp pain in specific regions of the head. Migraines are high-intensity headaches that can often lead to nausea and light sensitivity.

Treatment: Essential oils, like lavender, jasmine, rose, cedarwood, clary sage, fennel, and geranium all have calming properties which can provide relief from headaches. If the headache is due to an estrogen imbalance, then sandalwood oil can help to regulate the hormone.

Best practice: Sandalwood can be added to a cream or carrier oil and massaged onto the body or added to a bath. For relief from headaches, essential oils can be added to a cream or carrier oil and massaged into the temples, middle of the forehead, neck, and shoulders for relief. Diffusion and spraying a linen spray onto bedding before sleep can also help to relieve a headache.

Tips and tricks: If you are on-the-go, use the dry evaporation method and take a few deep breaths of lavender oil. However, when it comes to headaches, it is important not to go overboard with essential oils because continuous and excessive exposure to these strong and healing scents can cause headaches.

Heart Rate

Definition: Heart rate refers to the number of times the heart beats in a minute. A normal heart rate is between 60 and 100 beats. Anything below or above that is too fast or too slow (this refers to the resting rate of the heart and not the heart rate during or after exercise). The causes of a fast heart rate, also known as tachycardia, may include anxiety, high levels of estrogen, and stress. The causes of a slow heart rate, known as bradycardia, may be caused by hypothyroidism. It is important to note that you may have a naturally fast or slow heart rate and changes in this heart rate should be noted.

Symptoms: The symptoms of a fast heart rate can include palpitations, irregular heartbeat, and lightheadedness. Conversely, the symptoms of a slow heart rate can include fatigue and dizziness.

Treatment: Essential oils can help to ground you if you are experiencing a fast heart rate. Bergamot has been said to lower the heart rate, and frankincense and lavender oil can be used to calm the body and heart. Alternatively, grapefruit oil and orange oil can be used to energize the body. Rose geranium oil can be used to manage symptoms caused by hypothyroidism and balance the thyroid gland. Sandalwood oil can help to regulate and balance hormones secreted by the ovaries (i.e., estrogen).

Best practice: Add a few drops to a diffuser or use the dry evaporation method to return your heart rate to a normal rate quickly and effectively.

Tips and tricks: In the case of anxiety and increased heart rate due to stress and anxiety, carry an *emergency stress kit* with you at all times. Use some extra essential oil bottles that you may have lying around and create a mixture that relaxes you. Rose, lavender, and jasmine are great oils to use for this purpose. Add a few extra cotton balls and a small face cloth to the kit.

High Blood Pressure

Definition: High blood pressure, also known as hypertension, occurs when the blood that moves through the arteries is too forceful. Hypertension can be caused by stress, an unbalanced diet, excess growth hormones, and imbalances in the adrenal and pituitary glands.

Symptoms: Sometimes high blood pressure does not have any noticeable symptoms, which is what makes it so dangerous. Often, people realize they have high blood pressure too late and have already been diagnosed with high cholesterol or diabetes. This can be avoided by eating healthily, living a balanced life, and visiting the doctor regularly. Some symptoms may include fatigue, headaches, dizziness, and impaired vision.

Treatment: Grapefruit, sandalwood, and ylang-ylang oil all have properties that can lower blood pressure. Lemon oil can help to support and balance the adrenal gland while cedarwood oil can bring balance to the pituitary gland. To fight symptoms of fatigue, orange and grapefruit oil can energize the mind and body and lavender oil can be used to treat headaches.

Best practice: To access the pituitary glands, add a few drops of cedarwood oil diluted in a cream or carrier oil and massage into the temples, neck, and shoulders. To help lower blood pressure, grapefruit, sandalwood, and ylang-ylang can be added to a diffuser or inhaled through the dry evaporation method.

Tips and tricks: Diet and stress often have an influence over blood pressure. To ensure you are getting the most out of essential oil therapy, make sure you are eating enough vegetables, staying away from foods that are high in fat, and making an effort to reduce stress levels.

Inflammation

Definition: Inflammation is the body's immune response to external factors inside of the body. The body produces more white blood cells for protection which, in turn, leads to inflammation

Symptoms: The symptoms of inflammation manifest as swelling, redness, pain, and heat. Inflammation can occur almost anywhere in the body. Some digestive issues may be caused by inflammation and physical injury also leads to inflammation.

Treatment: Almost all essential oils have anti-inflammatory properties. However, some are more effective than others. To relieve symptoms of inflammation, try using thyme, chamomile, clove, and rosemary oil for the best results.

Best practice: The best way to reduce inflammation is to apply a warm compress soaked in water and a few drops of essential oil to the affected area. If you are experiencing general stiffness or inflammation of any kind, taking a warm bath with a few drops of essential oil can help to soothe the pain and increase circulation to evenly disperse the white blood cells.

Tips and tricks: While a warm compress will probably do the trick, massaging essential oils that are diluted in a carrier oil or cream in a circular motion can also help to relieve pain and reduce inflammation. For physical injury, eucalyptus oil can be applied to the affected area for optimal relief.

Infertility

Definition: Infertility refers to the inability of both men and women to produce offspring. Infertility can be caused by various issues, including hormonal imbalance. If progesterone, estrogen, follicle-stimulating hormone, and testosterone levels are insufficient or excessive, then infertility can occur.

Symptoms: Symptoms of infertility may include, but are not limited to irregular menstrual cycles, weight gain, hair loss, baldness, and pain during sex.

Treatment: Sandalwood oil can have balancing effects on the hormones produced by the ovaries (mainly estrogen and progesterone) while rosemary oil can be used to balance testosterone levels.

Best practice: Add a few drops of essential oil to a cream or carrier oil and apply to the body. A few drops of essential oil can also be added to a bath so that the whole body can absorb the effects of the essential oil.

Tips and tricks: Antioxidants can help to improve fertility. Black pepper, fennel, and mandarin oil are high in antioxidants and can be diffused into a room or inhaled with the dry evaporation method to enhance fertility.

Irregular Periods

Definition: Irregular periods refer to inconsistent and abnormal menstrual cycles. Irregular periods can be caused by stress, diet, medication, or an imbalance in estrogen and progesterone.

Symptoms: The symptoms of irregular periods are abnormal and inconsistent bleeding, menstrual cramps, and spotting between periods.

Treatment: Sandalwood oil helps to balance progesterone and estrogen levels. Clary sage can also be used to balance hormones.

Best practice: Add a few drops of essential oil to a warm compress and apply to the abdominal area. This can help relieve some symptoms caused by irregular periods and help to balance hormones.

These oils can also be added to a cream, carrier oil, or bath.

Tips and tricks: For an extra boost, ginger and cinnamon oil can also be used to regulate menstruation. Add a few drops to a diffuser and enjoy the warmth these oils have to offer.

Muscle Weakness

Definition: Muscle weakness refers to a decrease in muscle mass and strength. Muscle weakness can be caused by low levels of cortisol.

Symptoms: The symptoms of muscle weakness include fatigue, difficulty moving, lifting, or standing.

Treatment: Cassia and clary sage oil aid in circulation, which can help blood move through your body and strengthen muscles. Clary sage oil and basil oil can also help to balance hormones produced by the adrenal glands. Orange and grapefruit oil can energize the body and relieve fatigue.

Best practice: Add a few drops of clary sage, cassia, and basil oil to a cream or carrier oil and massage the body to stimulate blood circulation. These oils can also be added to a bath. Add a few drops of orange and grapefruit oil to a diffuser and take several deep breaths to promote circulation.

Tips and tricks: In most cases, essential oils decrease the level of cortisol in the body. In the case of muscle weakness, the levels are already too low.

Sandalwood can balance testosterone levels in the body and this balancing may result in increased muscle mass which can reduce muscle weakness.

Polycystic Ovary Syndrome (PCOS)

Definition: PCOS is a hormonal condition which results in cysts forming on the ovaries. PCOS is still being studied and there is a lot that is unknown about this disorder. However, it is known that the cysts formed on the ovaries have far-reaching effects on the female body.

Symptoms: Some symptoms of this disorder may include, but are not limited to, irregular periods, increased amounts of androgen which results in hair growth, acne, and hair loss. PCOS may lead to infertility, anxiety, depression, endometrial cancer, and high blood pressure.

Treatment: While essential oil therapy may not be able to cure PCOS, it can help to ease the symptoms. Many oils can ease feelings of anxiety and depression, like lavender and clary sage. Sandalwood oil can help to balance the androgen levels in the body, thus easing the symptoms of acne, and hair loss and growth. Acne can be treated with tea tree oil. Clary sage oil can also be used to level out estrogen and bring balance to the hormones secreted by the ovaries.

Best practice: For feelings of anxiety and depression, diffuse a few drops of lavender oil into the space you are in. To balance androgen levels in the body, add a few drops of sandalwood to a bath or to a cream or carrier oil and apply directly to the affected areas. Tea tree oil should be diluted with a cream and applied to acne to ease redness and reduce scarring. Clary sage oil can be diffused or added to a warm compress and applied to the abdominal area.

Tips and tricks: If you are suffering from PCOS, you might find that you experience other symptoms of hormonal imbalance. Luckily, the guide provided can help you to identify your symptoms and the oils that should be used to relieve these symptoms.

Skin Issues

Definition: Skin issues can refer to quite a few different conditions. Many of these conditions will be discussed individually and, therefore, this section will deal with uneven pigment, sunspots, and general discoloration. These conditions occur when there is too much or too little melanin being produced in certain areas of the skin.

Symptoms: The symptoms of overproduction or underproduction of melanin may include spots of discoloration on the skin. This can result in areas of skin that are lighter or darker than the rest of the skin.

Treatment: While there is often very little that can be done to help lighter spots, darker spots can be evened and reduced with frankincense oil, geranium oil, and tea tree oil. This is because these oils stimulate collagen production which reduces the effects of uneven pigmentation.

Best practice: Add a few drops of the essential oil to a carrier oil or cream and apply daily to the affected areas.

Tips and tricks: The process may take some time, so be careful not to try to speed it up by using too much oil or applying cream several times a day. Remember, moderation is key.

Swollen Ankles

Definition: Swollen ankles are caused by increased fluid in the leg, ankle, and foot areas. This can be caused by a variety of catalysts, like pregnancy, immobility, unbalanced diet, or poor circulation. Also, hormonal occurrences like menopause and hyperthyroidism can lead to fluid retention which in turn causes swollen ankles.

Symptoms: Swelling, inflammation, and pain can be symptoms of swollen ankles.

Treatment: Lavender, chamomile, eucalyptus, frankincense, and copaiba oil all have anti-inflammatory properties which can help to ease the swelling and pain caused by swollen ankles. However, with regard to swollen ankles caused by hormonal imbalances, it is necessary to treat the effect as well as the cause. In these cases, clary sage oil and frankincense oil are the most effective in treating hormonal imbalance symptoms caused by menopause and thyroid issues due to their anti-inflammatory, immune-boosting, and calming properties.

Best practice: Add a few drops to a cream or carrier oil and massage onto the ankles, legs, and feet. These oils can also be added to a bath or warm compress to reduce swelling and restore hormonal balance.

Tips and tricks: To help get rid of swelling, drink at least two liters of water a day. This might sound contradictory because the swelling is caused by water retention. However, keeping the body hydrated means it no longer has to store as much water and will, therefore, stop retaining excess amounts of water and aid in reducing the swelling.

Thyroid Issues

Definition: Hypothyroidism is when the thyroid gland does not make enough thyroid hormones, therefore, creating an imbalance. This imbalance can lead to Hashimoto's disease, which is an autoimmune condition that causes the body to attack its own thyroid gland. Hyperthyroidism occurs when the thyroid gland produces too much of the thyroid hormones, thus creating a hormonal imbalance. This can lead to Graves' disease which works in a similar way to Hashimoto's disease wherein the body attacks the thyroid gland.

Symptoms: The symptoms of hypothyroidism include tiredness, constipation, low bone density, high cholesterol, slow heart rate, and hair loss. Hashimoto's disease causes depression, constipation, loss in muscle mass, swelling, weight gain, and hair loss. While symptoms of hyperthyroidism include weight loss, heart palpitations, excessive sweating, mood swings, irregular periods, and insomnia. Graves' disease can cause anxiety, weight loss, and puffy eyes.

Treatment: Rose geranium, lemongrass, clary sage, and frankincense oil have been said to balance the hormones of the thyroid gland. Lavender oil can help to ease symptoms of anxiety and depression. Chamomile oil can be used to reduce inflammation and swelling while ginger and peppermint oil can help with hair loss symptoms.

Best practice: Add a few drops of essential oil to a cream or carrier oil and apply to the neck (where the thyroid gland is located). For inflammation, apply the cream to affected areas and massage the scalp with oil to stimulate hair growth.

Tips and tricks: Make sure your body gets enough rest and sleep. A balanced lifestyle can do wonders for an overactive or underactive thyroid.

Weight Gain

Definition: Weight gain refers to an increase in body mass. Weight gain can be due to muscle growth;

however, it can also be a result of overeating or hormonal imbalance. Treating weight gain is more challenging than meets the eye. There are many reasons for weight gain which could range anywhere from a tumor to menopause. For the purpose of this book, this section will explore the hormonal causes of weight gain. Hyper- and hypothyroidism are often leading causes of weight gain and so are increased levels of cortisol. Also, having too much estrogen, progesterone, or testosterone can result in weight gain.

Symptoms: The symptoms of weight gain include extra body mass.

Treatment: Fennel and grapefruit oil have appetite suppressing qualities and can help in reducing the extent of weight gain and aid in weight loss. Using oils like lavender and jasmine will help to lower the levels of cortisol in the body, aiding in weight loss, given that the main cause of weight gain is stress. Sandalwood helps to even out progesterone and estrogen, which can help with weight loss and rosemary oil is good for balancing testosterone.

Best practice: For these oils to help with weight loss and reduce weight gain, they should be diffused in a room or inhaled using the dry evaporation method when you are experiencing cravings.

Tips and tricks: If you are feeling fatigued or tired and don't have the energy to go for a walk or do some exercise, taking a few deep breaths of orange oil will energize and refocus your brain and body.

Chapter 8

Mental Symptoms of Hormonal Imbalance

Anxiety

Definition: Anxiety is a mental disorder that manifests in feelings of worry, stress, and fear. There are many different causes of anxiety, such as trauma, medication, and stress.

Symptoms: The symptoms of anxiety include, but are not limited to, dissociation, fidgeting, zoning-out, panic, worry, fear, sweating, hypervigilance, inability to focus, irritability, and mood swings. Anxiety can lead to panic attacks, and other mental health disorders.

Treatment: While anxiety often has deeper causes that need to be dealt with professionally, essential oils can help relieve the symptoms of anxiety. Lavender, chamomile, rose, jasmine, black pepper, cinnamon, clove, angelica, and quite a few other oils all have calming properties. Because anxiety is a personal struggle, finding an oil that works for you is crucial. Most essential oils have calming and soothing properties, so choosing an oil that eases your anxiety in intense moments can help to alleviate your symptoms of anxiety.

Best practice: To help with grounding when experiencing severe anxiety, use the dry evaporation method and take a few deep breaths until the feelings of panic subside. Essential oils can also be diffused into the room to promote calmness and a few drops can be added to a shower or bath before bed to promote sleep and relaxation. Add a few drops of essential oil to a cream or carrier oil and rub into the temples and middle of the forehead.

Tips and tricks: While applying cream, or taking a bath, use breathing exercises to calm the mind and body.

Brain Fog

Definition: Brain fog refers to an inability to focus, concentrate, recall memories, or think clearly. Brain fog can be caused by many different issues, such as imbalanced diet, anxiety, depression, lack of sleep, or thyroid issues.

Symptoms: Brain fog inhibits the ability to concentrate. This may lead to confusion, disorientation, and difficulty interpreting situations.

Treatment: Oils like orange, lemon, lemongrass, peppermint, grapefruit, and mandarin can energize the brain and clear up brain fog by improving concentration and focus. Rose oil can be used to relieve stress which could be causing the brain fog, and sandalwood oil can balance the thyroid gland.

Best practice: Take a few deep breaths of orange oil using the dry evaporation method or add a few drops to a diffuser and feel the fog lift from your brain.

Tips and tricks: Exercise can be a great way to supplement essential oils as a treatment for brain fog. Get up, and get your blood flowing. Along with a good whiff of orange oil, you will be focused in no time.

Cognitive Issues

Definition: Cognitive issues refer to problems with the brain and its thinking capacity. These issues can range from brain fog to impaired memory to lack of concentration. Cognitive issues can be caused by a wide range of hormonal imbalances and disorders in the body including high blood pressure, hypothyroidism, or diabetes. They can also be caused by infections and tumors.

Symptoms: The symptoms may include difficulty focusing, having a limited attention span, difficulty processing information, mood swings, hallucinations, an inability to recall memories, and trouble processing emotions. These can lead to feelings of frustration.

Treatment: Due to the levels of frustration being experienced, finding relaxation and calm is crucial. Therefore, lavender, rose, cinnamon, clove, or jasmine oil are recommended to relieve the stress and anxiety surrounding the cognitive issues. Once a relaxed state is achieved, it is time to refocus and energize the brain with lemon, lemongrass, lime, orange, mandarin, peppermint, grapefruit, and spearmint oil. Treating the causes requires an array of oils. For hypothyroidism, clary sage and frankincense oil can be used to balance the hormones of the thyroid gland. For diabetes, cassia oil can be used to regulate blood sugar levels. Sandalwood and ylang-ylang oil can help to lower blood pressure.

Best practice: The best methods to ease symptoms of cognitive issues are dry evaporation and diffusion.

Tips and tricks: A suggested practice for relieving cognitive issues and the symptoms that accompany them is to start by relaxing. Add a few drops of lavender oil to a bath and carrier oil and massage the temples, neck, and shoulders while in the bath. Take the night to "stop thinking." Don't do anything, like work or planning, that requires too much mental exertion. The next day, when you are feeling relaxed and your brain has had some time to decompress, it is time to start the energizing process. Diffuse a few drops of grapefruit oil into your house or workplace three times a day for 30 minutes at a time. Depending on the cause of the cognitive issues, alternate between oils that treat the symptoms and oils that treat the cause.

Depression

Definition: Depression is a mental health disorder which affects mood by reducing levels of serotonin and dopamine in the brain and body. Depression can be caused by hormonal imbalances that occur during and after pregnancy, during menopause, and during puberty. Depression can also be caused by a hormonal imbalance in the thyroid gland.

Symptoms: The symptoms include, but are not limited to, mood swings, fatigue, apathy, loss of interest, insomnia, anxiety, inability to care for oneself, and changes in appetite.

Treatment: Dealing with depression is extremely challenging. It is hard to treat because it requires a lot of effort from the person experiencing the depression. This can be difficult when even something as simple as getting out of bed can feel impossible. While essential oils probably won't cure depression and right the wrongs in the world, they can give you the boost you need to get up out of bed and go see a doctor or psychologist or get yourself to work. Frankincense and rose geranium can be used to regulate thyroid imbalances while lavender, jasmine, rose, and bergamot can improve mood. Orange, grapefruit, lemon, and mandarin oil can stimulate the brain and body and reduce feelings of apathy and fatigue.

Best practice: Add a few drops of essential oils to a diffuser for a full-body aromatherapy experience and get all of the nerves and neurons in the body and brain working. Taking a few deep breaths of essential oils using the dry evaporation method can be useful when experiencing severe feelings of depression. This method can act as a *restart* button for the brain and body.

Tips and tricks: Clary sage, jasmine, and lavender all have antidepressant properties and can be mixed together for maximum effectiveness. When using essential oils to treat the symptoms of depression, it is important to associate the oil with something positive. For example, if you spritz the clary sage, lavender, and jasmine mixture into a room or add a few drops to a diffuser, try to do something positive like get out of bed or make a snack. Soon, the brain will associate this smell with action and self-care and the process will become more productive and joyful.

Difficulty Concentrating

Definition: Difficulty concentrating refers to an inability to focus on a task for an extended period of time without getting distracted. A lack of concentration inhibits the ability to grasp information effectively.

Symptoms: The symptoms include getting distracted easily, being unable to retain or recall information or make decisions.

Treatment: Peppermint, spearmint, rosemary, orange, and grapefruit oil can be effective in refocusing the brain and concentrating on one task.

Best practice: Add a few drops of oil to a diffuser or take a few deep breaths using the dry evaporation method for a quick hit to the system.

Tips and tricks: In severe cases where concentrating is impossible, it is okay to take a break. Either go exercise and give your mind a break or rub some jasmine oil (diluted in a cream or carrier oil) on your temples while you sit outside and get some fresh air. You will feel refreshed and ready to concentrate.

Hyperglycemia

Definition: Hyperglycemia is used to refer to high blood sugar levels in the body. High blood sugar does not always lead to diabetes but can still have harmful effects on the body.

Symptoms: Symptoms experienced may include nausea, difficulty concentrating, dizziness, headache, and increased thirst (dry mouth).

Treatment: Cassia oil can be used to regulate blood sugar levels in the body and chamomile and ginger oil can be used to treat the symptoms that accompany hyperglycemia.

Best practice: Add a few drops of Cassia oil to a cream or carrier oil and apply to the body. Add chamomile and ginger oil to a warm compress and place on the forehead to relieve symptoms of dizziness, nausea, and headaches.

Tips and tricks: Exercising is a great way to lower blood sugar levels in the body. Take a few deep breaths of cassia oil using the dry evaporation method and go for a run or do some yoga. You will feel better in no time, and so will your pancreas.

Low Energy

Definition: Low energy, fatigue, or tiredness refers to a lack of energy and a desire to rest or sleep, even after a full night's rest or while doing simple, everyday tasks.

Symptoms: Symptoms of fatigue and low energy include weakness, an inability to concentrate, a feeling of heaviness and strain to keep the body upright, mood swings, and dizziness.

Treatment: Orange, cinnamon, grapefruit, and lemon oil can be used to energize the brain and body.

Best practice: Add a few drops of oil to a diffuser or use the dry evaporation method to increase and maintain energy levels.

Tips and tricks: Stay away from oils that make you feel calm as they could make you feel even more tired. These include lavender, chamomile, rose, and jasmine. Stick to bright, refreshing oils that can uplift your mood and increase energy levels.

Memory Loss

Definition: Memory loss is when you struggle to recall memories. These can be short-term or long-term memories and can be caused by hormonal imbalances during menopause and pregnancy. It often arises due to a lack of estrogen.

Symptoms: The symptoms include forgetfulness, difficulty solving problems, and confusion.

Treatment: Clary sage oil can help to regulate levels of estrogen in the body. Memory loss can be difficult to treat; therefore, treating the symptoms is more realistic when it comes to holistic healing. Orange, grapefruit, mandarin, and peppermint oil can be used to energize and refocus the brain. Lavender and chamomile oil can be used to calm the brain and reduce frustration. Rosemary oil has been shown to improve memory.

Best practice: Add a few drops of oil to a diffuser or take a few deep breaths of the oil using the dry evaporation method.

Tips and tricks: Sometimes, certain smells can trigger certain memories or emotions. Try using scents to trigger memory.

Mood Swings

Definition: Mood swings refer to the abnormal and abrupt fluctuations in emotional and mental states. Mood swings can be caused by hormonal imbalances, mainly by fluctuations of estrogen levels. Excess levels of testosterone in the body can also cause mood swings.

Symptoms: The symptoms include irregular moods, quick changes in mood (going from happy to angry in a matter of seconds), and intense emotions and feelings.

Treatment: Sandalwood oil helps to regulate testosterone in the body, while clary sage helps to regulate levels of estrogen. These can be used to treat the causes of mood swings. To treat the symptoms, oils such as rose, chamomile, basil, peppermint, and jasmine can be used to relieve symptoms of mood swings and neutralize moods.

Best practice: Use the dry evaporation method when experiencing extreme changes in mood. Add a few drops to a diffuser for long-term relief from mood swings.

Tips and tricks: Mood swings happen quickly and can be challenging to identify when they occur. In these situations, breathing exercises as well as grounding and mindfulness exercises (along with the use of essential oils) can be useful in stabilizing moods.

Menopause

Definition: Menopause refers to the change in hormones (a decrease in reproductive hormones) in a woman between the ages of 40 and 50. When menopause starts, menstruation stops and progesterone and estrogen are no longer produced in large quantities. Pregnancy is no longer possible.

Symptoms: The symptoms of menopause include, but are not limited to, vaginal dryness, hot flashes, insomnia, mood swings, fatigue, anxiety, and a lowered sex drive.

Treatment: Due to its ability to regulate estrogen levels in the body, clary sage oil can be effective in lessening the effects of menopause. Ultimately, menopause will occur, but reducing the effects of the symptoms can bring great relief. Lavender and rose oil can help with insomnia and anxiety. Jasmine oil can help to increase sex drive. Lemon oil can reduce fatigue. Peppermint and eucalyptus oil can be used to limit the effects of a hot flash.

Best practice: Clary sage should be diffused into a space for maximum effectiveness. As for the other symptoms, lavender oil can be added to a cream or carrier oil and massaged into the temples or added to a bath. Jasmine oil can be added to a cream or carrier oil and massaged onto the body and added to a linen spray to be sprayed on bedsheets. Peppermint oil can be added to a cold compress to relieve the effects of a hot flash.

Tips and tricks: Menopause is about adjustment. It might not be fun, but it will pass. Maintaining a healthy lifestyle in conjunction with essential oil therapy will get you through the worst of it.

Sex Drive

Definition: The sex drive refers to an individual's desire to engage in sexual activity. Loss of a sex drive can be due to many factors, such as stress, anxiety, and relationship stress, but it can also be due to decreased levels of testosterone and estrogen in the body.

Symptoms: No desire or interest engaging in sexual activities.

Treatment: Clary sage oil can balance levels of estrogen in the body, while sandalwood can help to regulate testosterone. Jasmine oil has been known to increase the sex drive, as have basil, copaiba, ginger, and rose oil.

Best practice: Add a few drops of oil to a diffuser or add to a linen spray to increase sex drive.

Tips and tricks: If you are struggling with a loss of your sex drive, it may also be due to increased levels of stress. Add some jasmine oil to a bath and take a second to relax and unwind.

Sleep Issues

Definition: Insomnia refers to the inability to sleep, as well as difficulty getting to and staying asleep.

Symptoms: Symptoms of insomnia include the inability to concentrate, fatigue, drowsiness, and depression.

Treatment: Angelica, cedarwood, bergamot, frankincense, clary sage, jasmine, lavender, and chamomile oil all have calming properties that aid in sleep.

Best practice: Add a few drops to a linen spray and spray onto the bed several minutes before getting into bed. A few drops can also be added to a warm compress and placed on the head.

Tips and tricks: Make sure that you are not exposed to light before bed (i.e., the television or your phone) as the light tricks your mind into thinking it is daytime, which makes the process of falling asleep more challenging.

Stress

Definition: Stress is a feeling of emotional or physical tension, worry, or fear that leads to mental and physical distress.

Symptoms: The symptoms of stress include depression, muscle tightness, headaches, anxiety, insomnia, mood swings, and feelings of worry.

Treatment: Lavender, rose, jasmine, frankincense, chamomile, and clary sage have calming properties that can help you to unwind and relax.

Best practice: Add a few drops to a diffuser and let the aroma permeate the room. Add a few drops to a cream or carrier oil and massage onto the body. Oils can also be added to showers and baths for maximum relaxation.

Tips and tricks: If you experience stress-induced muscle tightness and soreness, add some eucalyptus oil to a bath or warm compress to reduce inflammation and pain.

Chapter 9

Other Symptoms of Hormonal Imbalance

Aging

Definition: Aging refers to the process of getting older. Essential oils can help to slow the aging process through holistic healing.

Symptoms: The process of aging comes with weakened bones, low bone density, cognitive issues, skin issues, and a lack of a sex drive. While some conditions are more serious than others, some can be helped, and even prevented, with essential oils.

Treatment: Jasmine oil can increase the sex drive. Patchouli and tea tree oil can be used for skincare as they promote collagen production and, therefore, lower the risk and presence of wrinkles. A fresh burst of orange oil in the morning can wake the brain and help with memory and other cognitive issues while thyme and rosemary oil can help strengthen bones.

Best practice: Add some jasmine oil to a diffuser or linen spray to boost your sex drive. Tea tree oil and patchouli oil can be added to a cream or carrier oil and applied to the skin daily. Orange oil can be added to a diffuser to keep energy levels high and rosemary and thyme oil can be added to a warm compress and applied to affected areas.

Tips and tricks: Aging can be a difficult thing to accept—it is inevitable. However, that does not mean that you can't use essential oils to cheat the system a little. Essential oils and holistic healing can delay the aging process by keeping you young and full of life.

Body Odor

Definition: Body odor refers to the body's natural scent that may be considered unpleasant due to the bacteria that breaks down proteins from sweat.

Symptoms: An unpleasant smell from the skin.

Treatment: Cypress and tea tree oil have been known to contain unpleasant smells due to their antibacterial properties. These essential oils kill the bacteria found on the surface of this skin, therefore, reducing the chances of bacteria interacting with and breaking down sweat.

Best practice: Add a few drops to a cream or carrier oil and apply to the areas where body odor is most noticeable.

Tips and tricks: The great thing about using essential oils as a deodorant is that you will not only *not* smell bad, you'll smell great. Add a few drops of jasmine or angelica oil for a more perfumed scent.

Circulation

Definition: Circulation is a very important part of regulating temperatures and ensuring the health and function of the body. Poor circulation refers to the inadequacy of blood circulation in the body. Low levels of estrogen can cause poor blood circulation.

Symptoms: Poor circulation can often lead to always having cold hands and feet because the blood doesn't quite reach the extremities fast enough. Symptoms may include cramping, swelling, and pain.

Treatment: Clary sage oil can be used to regulate the levels of estrogen in the body if that is what is causing poor circulation. Cassia, clary sage, rosemary, and grapefruit oil can all help to improve blood circulation. Angelica, sage, and jasmine oil have antispasmodic properties which can help to reduce the effects and frequency of spasms and cramps in the muscles. They can also be applied to reduce swelling and pain.

Best practice: Add a few drops to a cream or carrier oil and massage the skin in a linear motion to get the blood flowing to the extremities. A few drops can also be added to a warm compress to increase blood circulation in the body.

Tips and tricks: Improving circulation is about getting blood flowing. Try exercising for a few minutes before applying a warm compress or massaging the arms and legs to get a head start on the blood flow.

Endometriosis

Definition: This is when the lining of the uterus (which is supposed to grow inside of the uterus) grows on the outside. Endometriosis can be caused by excess levels of estrogen in the body.

Symptoms: The symptoms of endometriosis include pain in the lower back and abdomen, as well as during sex. Other symptoms that can be experienced are irregular periods, constipation, cramping, and infertility.

Treatment: Clary sage oil can be used to regulate estrogen levels. Lavender, jasmine, and clary sage oil can be used to relieve cramping and pain. Peppermint oil can be used to relieve digestive issues.

Best practice: Add a few drops of these oils to a warm compress and apply to the affected areas (mainly the lower back and abdominal areas). Clary sage oil can also be added to a bath or diffused into a room.

Tips and tricks: Heat helps to relieve the symptoms of endometriosis, which is why a warm compress can be useful. Oils, like cinnamon and clove, can be useful in reducing inflammation and treating cramps.

Hair Loss

Definition: Hair loss refers to the loss of hair from the scalp and other areas of the body.

Symptoms: Symptoms include the loss and thinning of hair on the body.

Treatment: Ginger, peppermint, rosemary, cedarwood, and thyme oil can all be used to promote hair growth. They have heating properties and, therefore, stimulate hair follicles and increase blood flow to targeted areas.

Best practice: Add a few drops of essential oil to a cream or carrier oil and massage into the scalp or affected areas for a few minutes every day.

Tips and tricks: For extra hair growth, add a few drops of essential oil to shampoo or conditioner and massage into the scalp.

Itching

Definition: Itching is a sensation that involves a desire to scratch parts of the body that feel itchy. This can be due to dry skin, rashes, ingrown hairs, or hair growth (after shaving or waxing).

Symptoms: Scratching the irritated and itchy spots may lead to redness, scratches, flaky skin, inflammation, and small bumps on the surface of the skin.

Treatment: Clove oil has been shown to relieve chronic itching. Patchouli, rose, and ylang-ylang oil have hydrating properties which can help to bring moisture to the skin and reduce itching.

Best practice: Add a few drops of oil to a cream or carrier oil and apply to the affected areas. If itching is experienced throughout the body, add a few drops of water to a cold bath and submerge the skin in the water to hydrate the skin and relieve inflammation.

Tips and tricks: Itching can be extremely annoying and frustrating. Applying a cold compress can relieve itching because it reduces inflammation and therefore reduces general irritation. Just resist the urge to scratch.

Osteoporosis

Definition: Osteoporosis refers to the weakening of bones. This often affects the back which leads to a slight curve in the spine. It also increases the chances of bone fractures.

Symptoms: The symptoms of osteoporosis include pain and bone fractures.

Treatment: Thyme and rosemary oil are effective in treating osteoporosis. Eucalyptus oil and frankincense can help to reduce pain and inflammation.

Best practice: Add a few drops of oil to a warm compress and apply to the affected areas. A few drops can also be added to a warm bath to help relieve symptoms.

Tips and tricks: Thyme and rosemary (in herb form) can be added to meals or ingested in supplement form for an extra dose of natural healing.

Chapter 10

Other Important Ways to Balance Hormones

Essential oils are dynamic and multifaceted tools that can be used for holistic healing. However, I am sure that you have come to realize that using essential oils in conjunction with other holistic forms of healing can only benefit you. Similarly, when you get sick and decide to see a doctor, they do not only prescribe medicine and send you on your way. They give you medicine and tell you to get plenty of rest, eat well, and take the medicine according to the instructions. Yes, the medication will still be effective if you neglect to follow the rest of the instructions, but the road to recovery is shorter if you give your body the rest and nutrients it needs. Essential oil therapy works in the same way, especially when it comes to treating and relieving the symptoms of hormonal imbalances. This chapter will provide a guide on additional holistic therapies and habits that can be used to treat hormonal imbalance. Factors like diet, body movement, and supplements can amplify the effects of essential oil therapy. Plus, food and supplements can target specific hormonal imbalance symptoms. For example, if you suffer from irregular periods due to an estrogen imbalance, then eating foods and using essential oils that balance the estrogen levels in the body is a great way to ensure speedy and natural healing.

Diet

While essential oils are a great way to balance hormones and relieve symptoms of stress and anxiety, there are other ways to supplement essential oil therapy to get the best results. It is not only about getting the best results, it is about feeling the best you can by living a healthy and balanced life. Here is a guide to using food to restore and maintain hormone balance:

- Regulating estrogen

Sesame seeds, chickpeas, garlic, and dried fruit contain compounds called phytestrogens. These compounds are similar to the estrogen that is in the body. Eating these foods can help to lower blood pressure, increase circulation, and help with the symptoms of pregnancy and menopause. However, if you are experiencing hormonal imbalance symptoms caused by an excess of estrogen in the body, then these foods should be avoided as they can increase estrogen levels. Unlike essential oils which regulate imbalances, using food to balance hormones tends to go one way. Levels of estrogen cannot be decreased by eating foods that contain phytestrogens. These foods will only increase estrogen and, therefore, need to be consumed in moderation. Excess levels of estrogen can lead to high blood pressure, endometriosis, mood swings, memory loss, irregular periods, weight gain, and infertility. Even if the body lacks estrogen, moderation is important. Eating these foods in smaller quantities will be more beneficial.

- Thyroid gland

In the case of hypothyroidism, eating foods that contain iodine (fish, salt, and seaweed) can balance the thyroid hormones. The thyroid requires iodine for hormone production. Hypothyroidism occurs when there is not enough of the thyroid hormones being produced and, therefore, increasing your iodine intake can increase hormone production and bring balance to the thyroid and body. Symptoms of hypothyroidism include tiredness, constipation, low bone density, and high cholesterol. To help relieve these symptoms, eating vegetables like kale and spinach can add fiber to the diet and reduce fatigue. Oats and nuts can lower cholesterol levels and increasing the intake of calcium can help to strengthen bones.

Hyperthyroidism works in the opposite way. Because the thyroid is producing too much of the thyroid hormones, you want to reduce the intake of iodine to curb the production of hormones. Therefore, it is best to stay away from iodized salt, fish, bananas, and seaweed. Eating foods that are low in iodine can slow the production of hormones and reduce the effects of hyperthyroidism. These foods include egg whites (try to avoid egg yolks), vegetables (like cabbage and broccoli), and oats. Replacing milk and other dairy products with non-dairy products like almond milk can also reduce iodine intake.

- Inflammation

While essential oils have you covered on the anti-inflammatory front, adding a few anti-inflammatory ingredients to your diet can only be beneficial. Inflammation can be reduced by eating vegetables, specifically tomatoes and leafy greens (like kale). Lemon, berries, avocado, and ginger can also be effective in reducing inflammation. Foods that contain high amounts of antioxidants often have anti-inflammatory properties. For external inflammation, like acne, itching, rashes, or redness, apply a warm compress with tea tree oil and have a bowl of berries. Treating inflammation externally and internally can help to relieve pain, discomfort, and redness faster.

- Gut health

Your gut is a microbiome. This means that it contains many different microorganisms, bacteria (both good and bad), and enzymes to maintain a healthy and balanced digestive system. The food going into the digestive system should be able to nourish the microbiome without causing too much disruption. Artificial and processed foods, as well as foods that are high in sugar, can throw off the natural microbes of the stomach and cause inflammation and irritation. To maintain gut health, fermented foods like kimchi, or substances like kefir and kombucha can help to restore *good* bacteria. Similarly, yogurt is also a good source of probiotics and can ease inflammation.

- Regulate testosterone

Regulating testosterone can take one of two roads. Either testosterone needs to be lowered or it needs to be increased. Foods that help to reduce the levels of testosterone in the body include foods that contain phytestrogens, such as sesame seeds, dried fruits, soy, and garlic. These foods can help to decrease the testosterone and increase the estrogen levels. When trying to increase testosterone, it is best to stay away from foods that contain large amounts of phytestrogen. Foods that help to increase testosterone include meat, egg yolks, oysters, and ginger. Vitamin D, proteins, and calcium. Therefore, foods that are high in vitamin D, proteins, and calcium can increase testosterone levels, prevent infertility, increase bone density and muscle mass, and help with the sex drive.

- Strengthen bones

Calcium is largely responsible for bone health and density. Milk, dairy products (like cheese and yogurt), tofu, and nuts are good sources of calcium. Vegetables also play an important role in strengthening and maintaining bones. Balancing estrogen levels in the body can also have a positive effect on bone growth and density; therefore, eating foods that contain phytestrogens can contribute to strengthening bones. Foods like sweet potatoes and spinach should be avoided as they can reduce calcium absorption.

- Hair and skin

Eating healthily can help to resolve skin issues like rashes, acne, and eczema, especially if the cause of these issues is dryness. To combat dry skin and dandruff, it is crucial to have a diet that is high in fat and antioxidants. Fish and nuts can hydrate the skin and scalp and combat dryness. Alternatively, if the skin is too oily, then these foods should be avoided. Foods like carrots and oats can nourish hair, promote hair growth, and prevent hair loss. Bananas can also help with eczema and skin irritation.

- Mental health

While depression and anxiety are psychological issues, certain foods can help to treat the symptoms that accompany these mental disorders. For example, anxiety promotes inflammation. Therefore, eating foods that reduce inflammation can help offset the effects of anxiety. Nuts, fruits, and foods high in antioxidants can reduce inflammation. The healthier your body, the easier it will be to handle anxiety and depression. Caffeine should be avoided to prevent increased heart rate and feelings of anxiety. For depression, fish, nuts, and spinach can help to improve your mood. However, similarly to essential oils, while eating healthily and using aromatherapy

184

can offset certain symptoms, it won't cure depression and anxiety, although that doesn't mean eating right and diffusing some lavender oil into your room won't help.

- Weight gain

Weight gain is often due to overeating. However, sometimes due to thyroid issues, an excess of estrogen and testosterone, or menopause, it doesn't matter how little you eat, weight gain feels inevitable. While using essential oils to suppress appetite and cravings, eating certain foods can also reduce the amount of weight gain. Foods like celery, kale, spinach, and broccoli are healthy, low calorie and fibrous, meaning that your body expends energy digesting them.

- Fatigue

Fatigue can be a debilitating symptom of hormonal imbalance. Try to avoid carbohydrates as they offer a short-lived burst of energy. It is better to eat proteins which offer a slow and consistent release of energy. Eating fruits and vegetables will also increase energy and reduce the symptoms of fatigue. Hydration is also a big factor in reducing tiredness. Make sure to drink enough water so that dehydration does not contribute to feelings of fatigue and tiredness.

- Sex drive

Foods that can improve a sex drive have aphrodisiac qualities. These include oysters, asparagus, figs, chocolate, and chilies. These foods also increase blood flow and can help with low sex drive and erectile dysfunction. Stay away from alcohol and carbohydrates as they will only weigh you down. Alcohol is a depressant and can reduce erectile function.

- High blood pressure

High blood pressure can have serious effects on your health, including heart disease and strokes. Similarly to how grapefruit essential oil can help to lower blood pressure, grapefruit and other citrus fruits can also lower blood pressure. It is best to avoid processed foods and foods that have a high fat content. Even if your blood pressure is too low and needs to be increased, avoiding processed food is still a good strategy. Instead, increase your intake of salt and drink more water.

Body Movement

Exercising is also a very effective way of balancing hormones on your journey to holistic healing. As you know, yoga is an effective tool for holistic healing and general balancing. However, there are other forms of body movement that can be beneficial to maintaining mental, physical, and spiritual balance. There are many kinds of body movement techniques available for you to learn and try and the movement that is the most comfortable for you is the one you should focus on. Yoga, Pilates, swimming, or any form of exercise can be beneficial in balancing hormones and making you feel better. Another form of holistic healing and exercise is known as Tai Chi.

Tai Chi is a Chinese martial art that has been practiced since the 15th century. It is used for defense and, similarly to yoga, can be used for meditation and health. It involves a series of movements that flow into one another. The principles of Tai Chi include "relaxation, grounding, presence, stance, structure, spirit, and intent" (Taiji Forum, n.d.). These principles allow for a balance between movement and meditation which are fundamental components of holistic healing. Tai Chi has been shown to reduce stress levels, improve sleep, and improve sex drive. Practices like Tai Chi can bring you closer to your body and make it easier to identify the wants and needs of the being. If you are in-tune with your body you will be able to know when something is off-balance.

Supplements

Sometimes diets don't give your body everything it needs. Perhaps you are a vegetarian or vegan and need to supplement your diet to make sure your body is balanced. Perhaps the hormonal imbalance you are experiencing requires a specific type of supplement. In these cases, supplements can be extremely useful in bringing balance to the body and in rectifying hormonal imbalance. Here are a few supplements that can help keep your hormones balanced:

1. Maca powder

Maca powder is made from the root of the maca plant. The root is dried and crushed into a fine powder and consumed. However, maca can also be cooked and added to a variety of different meals. It is a very versatile vegetable that is native to Peru. The powder can be found at any pharmacy or health store. Maca powder is famous for increasing the sex drive but it has many other benefits. This is because it has hormone-balancing properties which help to regulate the levels of estrogen and testosterone in the body. This means that maca powder can also help to lower blood pressure, reduce mood swings and the effects of menopause, help with endometriosis, and improve circulation. It also means that regulated testosterone levels can improve fertility, one's sex drive, help with androgen deficiency, improve bone density, and increase muscle mass. Maca powder can be added to smoothies, baked goods (like granola bars or cookies), porridge, or it can be taken as a supplement in tablet form. However, maca powder does not just work overnight so it is important to consume one to two teaspoons of maca powder daily for one to two months before the full benefits of the powder can be experienced.

2. Spirulina

Spirulina, unlike maca powder, is not a root or vegetable. It is algae that can be consumed by humans or animals and offers many health benefits. Spirulina is grown in freshwater, but is farmed in freshwater pools for commercial purposes. Spirulina comes in powder or tablet form and can be taken as a supplement or added to smoothies, juice, water, cooked with, added to oatmeal, or sprinkled on top of salad. It tastes better than maca powder so it can easily be added to snacks and meals. However, it will turn everything green, so if the idea of a dark green bowl of oatmeal does not appeal to you, maybe stick to smoothies. Spirulina has many hormone-balancing benefits, one of which is preventing the release of excess estrogen into the body. Having too much estrogen in the body can have inflammatory effects which lead to mood swings, high blood pressure, and increased menopause symptoms. Spirulina ensures that estrogen levels are regulated, therefore reducing the effects of inflammation on the body. Half a teaspoon to one teaspoon of spirulina can be taken daily. Spirulina also contains large amounts of vitamin E which can help to boost mood, reduce mood swings, and help with anxiety and depression.

3. Probiotics

Probiotics, similarly to spirulina, are naturally grown supplements. While spirulina is algae, probiotics consist of bacteria and yeast that help to regulate and maintain gut health. Probiotics regulate the bacteria balance of the body. If you are experiencing constipation, probiotics can ease this by targeting the harmful bacteria with *good* bacteria. Probiotics help with gut health, but they can also help regulate the bacteria in the mouth and vagina. They can help with yeast infections and using probiotics alongside lemongrass, thyme, and tea tree oil to treat oral and vaginal thrush can act as a natural treatment for candida. Probiotics can also be taken alongside peppermint oil to regulate the digestive system, treat irritable bowel syndrome, and reduce inflammation. Probiotics can be taken in tablet form daily to maintain gut health.

4. Zinc

Zinc is a mineral produced by the body that helps the immune system. It helps you to stay healthy and can be a useful supplement to take for colds and flu. It can be taken in tablet form and can also be found in medication. Zinc can increase the levels of testosterone in the body which can help with sex drive, muscle mass, bone density, and fertility. Zinc is also an important nutrient during pregnancy and is necessary for fetal growth. It can regulate levels of estrogen and progesterone in the body which is useful during pregnancy or menopause. Zinc can lower blood sugar levels and increase circulation in the body. However, it is also important to note that taking too much zinc can have adverse effects such as nausea, headaches, and cramps. To reap the full benefits of zinc it must be used in moderation. Unless otherwise recommended by a healthcare professional, avoid high doses of zinc and opt for a zinc supplement that is under 10mg. Try not to use zinc for extended periods of time as it can affect the way your body absorbs copper and should therefore be taken as a supplement once a week.

5. Vitamin D

Vitamin D is famous for its affiliation with the sun. While it is true that the sun can be a good source of vitamin D, there may be factors that prevent you from basking in the sun. Perhaps you live in a country that does not often have sun, or you find yourself indoors most of the time. Luckily, vitamin D can be taken daily in tablet form. Vitamin D helps the body absorb calcium which in turn strengthens bones. It is also an important element in fighting off illness. Vitamin D regulates estrogen levels which can reduce depression, mood swings, blood pressure, and improve circulation. Vitamin D deficiency can have debilitating effects on the body, leading to brittle and weak bones, fatigue, pain, and mood swings. This is why having enough vitamin D is essential to the healthy functioning of the body.

6. Calcium

Calcium is crucial to survival. Without calcium, bones and muscles would not have sufficient density (or any density for that matter) to keep the body healthy and alive. Calcium does not only strengthen bones and teeth but it also aids with blood clotting.

While blood clots can be life-threatening, the ability to clot makes it possible for wounds to heal. Without the ability to stop blood from leaving the body, a mere cut could lead to excessive amounts of blood loss. Therefore, calcium is necessary for living a healthy life. However, the body does not produce its own calcium and it must be supplemented. Calcium can be supplemented through food or taken in tablet form. The daily recommended intake is 500mg. However, this can increase with age to ensure sufficient bone and muscle strength. The parathyroid gland regulates calcium levels and balances estrogen, testosterone, and the growth hormone. These hormones all help with bone density, muscle mass, bone absorption, and general bone health. Vitamin D helps with the absorption of calcium and these vitamins can be taken together for optimal absorption. Calcium can prevent fractures, teeth problems, and reduce muscle pain.

7. Magnesium

Magnesium can balance blood sugar levels in the body as well as lower blood pressure. It is also important for muscle and bone health as it can build up protein in these areas. Magnesium also reduces inflammation which can help with many issues such as digestion, muscle soreness, and thyroid issues. It also produces and regulates estrogen and testosterone levels in the body which is why it is effective in lowering blood pressure. Having too little magnesium can cause fatigue and muscle weakness, making it difficult to do ordinary everyday tasks. Magnesium supplements should be taken daily to ensure the healthy functioning of the body. The recommended amount is between 300mg and 400mg of magnesium. Too much magnesium can cause digestive issues and nausea.

8. Omega 3

Omega 3s are fatty acids that are considered to be healthy fats that the body uses for energy. Omega 3 can be found in foods such as fish and seeds, but it can also be ingested as a supplement. Fish oil can also be used as an omega 3 supplement. Omega 3 can help with high blood pressure and also reduce the risk of heart disease. It also improves blood circulation which can help with erectile dysfunction or any other symptoms caused by poor circulation. It reduces inflammation and can help with acne. Omega 3 should be taken daily. The recommended dosage is between 1000mg and 3000mg a day. Even though omega 3 consists of fatty acids, it can actually aid in weight loss as it increases metabolic rates which means it helps your body burn energy faster. The more calories you burn, the more weight you can lose. Just remember to supplement omega 3 with healthy habits like a good diet and enough exercise. Grapefruit essential oil can also be used to suppress appetite and aid in weight loss. Omega 3 stimulates the brain and improves memory. It can be used in conjunction with rosemary essential oil to improve memory and reduce inflammation.

9. Vitamin B12

Vitamin B12 can either be taken as a supplement in tablet form or it can be injected into the body every few months. Between one microgram and three micrograms can be taken daily. Your body absorbs only what it needs and will excrete any excess vitamins in the body. Vitamin B12 regulates blood cells in the body, produces energy, and increases brain function. A deficiency in vitamin B12 can lead to anemia (the lack of red blood cells in the body), fatigue, constipation, lack of balance, and memory loss.

10. Selenium

Selenium is a mineral that regulates the metabolism and also benefits the thyroid gland. The body does not produce selenium and it must be added to the body. Selenium can be taken in supplement form between 70 and 200 micrograms daily. It has been shown to reduce the risk of heart disease because of its anti-inflammatory properties. Selenium is also rich in antioxidants which means that it is good for the hair, skin, and heart.

Essential oils can stand alone as a treatment therapy. However, if two heads are better than one, then the same applies to holistic healing. Essential oils provide a natural and organic alternative to pharmaceutical medicine. If plant extracts can have healing effects, then so, too, can plants. It also means that instead of ingesting essential oils, adding supplements and tailoring your diet to care for and bring balance to the body can help it experience external and internal healing. Consult a doctor on which supplements and dietary changes can benefit you the most. While selenium powder has many benefits to offer, you won't be able to reap these benefits if you are allergic to it. Blood tests and regular check-ups are a great way to keep up with how your body is functioning and what it needs.

Chapter 11

14-Day Detox Guide

Now that you have an understanding of essential oils, hormonal imbalance, and how the two interact to bring about holistic healing, it is time to put all of that information into practice. This two-week detox guide is intended to give you, regardless of your hormonal imbalance, a fresh and clean start to begin the healing process. Once the body and mind are detoxed, you can begin using specific essential oils to meet your healing needs. This guide can help you get into the habit of using essential oils and give you room for trial and error. You might find, during this 14-day period, that there are certain oils you don't like, and certain oils that are particularly effective. Find out what you like, what works for you, and use that information to aid in future healing. This guide will also give you a good starting collection of essential oils to have at your disposal. Before starting the 14-day detox, seek advice from a medical or healthcare professional to make sure you do not have any allergies or medical contradictions that may counteract the effect of the essential oils. Here is a checklist of the oils that will be required during the 14-days:

- ❑ Angelica
- ❑ Black pepper
- ❑ Cassia
- ❑ Cedarwood
- ❑ Chamomile
- ❑ Frankincense
- ❑ Grapefruit
- ❑ Ginger
- ❑ Jasmine
- ❑ Lavender
- ❑ Orange
- ❑ Rose
- ❑ Sandalwood
- ❑ Spearmint
- ❑ Ylang-ylang

Week 1

The first week is about detoxifying the body. It is about getting rid of all the toxins, processed foods, synthetic ingredients, and harmful bacteria in the body. While the detox is largely based on essential oils, it is also necessary to start implementing a healthy diet and exercise plan. This guide will provide structure in the mental and spiritual departments of holistic healing. It will help you to form habits and get you comfortable with practicing mindfulness and meditation. With regards to diet, follow a balanced diet plan and stay away from junk food. Try making smoothies, adding some maca powder to your daily routine, and start implementing supplements into your diet.

Day 1

Angelica, cassia, and cedarwood oil all have diuretic properties which make them perfect for detoxing. However, they won't all be used on the first day. To get started, add a few drops of orange oil to a diffuser or the walls of your shower and start the day with a burst of energy. At midday, add some ginger oil to a cotton ball and inhale using the dry evaporation method. This will start to promote gut health and get your body ready for the detoxifying process. In the evening, before bed, add a few drops of angelica oil to a cream or carrier oil and massage onto the skin. Angelica promotes urination and sweating which will help the body to begin the detoxification process. It is best to use this oil at night since the excess sweating and urination may be bothersome during the day. Day 1 is a great day to start practicing mindfulness and meditation. Start with a five-minute meditation and a 15-minute yoga session to get your blood flowing and your mind ready for the next 13 days.

Day 2

After a night of detoxifying, you might need a pick-me-up. Add some orange oil to a diffuser or the walls of the shower once again. At midday, use the dry evaporation method and take a few deep breaths of spearmint oil. Spearmint is a diuretic and has detoxifying properties. It also promotes focus and concentration. In the evening, add a few drops of cedarwood to a cream or carrier oil and massage into the temples and forehead. Cedarwood has detoxifying and relaxing properties and can help with insomnia. Continue to practice mindfulness and mediation in small bursts. Focus on the present moment and your breath when massaging the cedarwood oil onto the temples.

Day 3

Time to change things up a little. Start the day with a fresh burst of Angelica oil to promote relaxation and continue the detox. Add a few drops of Angelica oil to a diffuser while you get ready in the morning. At midday, add a few drops of lavender and rose oil to a diffuser. This will help with relaxation as the detoxifying process can be quite taxing on the body. In the evening, add a few drops of cassia oil to a bath. Not only will this help with relaxation and sleep, but cassia oil also has diuretic and laxative properties which allow for the detoxification process to progress. Take a moment in the day to practice a 10-minute meditation session and 20 minutes of yoga or exercise.

Day 4

Day 4 is about rest before the final detox stretch. Add a few drops of grapefruit oil to a room spray and spray into the room when you wake up. Grapefruit oil has mood-enhancing properties and will help you to start the day with energy and enthusiasm. At midday, add a few drops of rose oil to a diffuser while practicing a 15-minute meditation. In the evening, add some jasmine oil to a linen spray and spray onto bed sheets before sleeping.

Day 5

After a good night's rest and a day of relaxation, it is time to get back to detoxing. Add a few drops of angelica and cassia oil to a cream or carrier oil and massage onto the body. This will allow the skin to absorb the essential oils and detoxify for longer during the day. For this reason, using an oil at midday can be skipped. Instead, practice a 20-minute meditation and a 20-minute exercise session to get the blood flowing and speed up the metabolism. In the evening, add a mixture of rose, jasmine, and lavender oil to a diffuser and diffuse into the room before sleeping.

Day 6

Start the day with a few deep breaths of spearmint oil using the dry evaporation method. This will get the digestive system active and ready for the day ahead. At midday, add a few drops of ginger oil to hot water and proceed to steam for three to four minutes. This will clear the head and mind and stimulate the digestive system. Try to exercise either right before, or right after steaming to increase blood flow and absorption of the essential oil. In the evening, mix a few drops of chamomile and rose oil and spray onto linen before sleeping.

Day 7

The final day of serious detoxing and time to give your body a last dose of detoxifying goodness before moving on to the second half of the process. Add a few drops of orange and spearmint oil to the walls of the shower in the morning. At midday, mix angelica and cassia oil and diffuse into the room while completing a 25-minute meditation. Meditating for longer periods may be more challenging but it is important to focus on the rhythm of the breath and the scent of essential oils in the air. In the evening, add a few drops of chamomile oil to a cream or carrier oil and massage onto the skin. The process of detoxifying is now over and week 2 is about clearing the system in less literal ways.

Week 2

Week 1 prepared your mind, body, and soul through detoxing. Week 2 is about reducing inflammation, increasing relaxation, and starting a routine sleep schedule. This is where the full effects of essential oils are seen. Having a blank slate will give the essential oils a good basis to work with. If your body is full of toxins and harmful bacteria, then relaxing the mind, body, and soul, will be stunted and unsatisfying. Think of preparing for essential oil therapy as walking through a forest. It is getting dark and you have to make it to the top of the hill soon, otherwise, you will miss the sunset. If the path you are walking is filled with rocks, fallen trees, and an array of different obstacles, it is going to take longer to walk up the hill and you will most likely miss the sunset. However, if the path is clear, then you will be able to effortlessly walk up the hill and view the sunset in peace. Similarly, if healing is the goal and essential oil therapy is the path, if the path is encumbered by heart disease, toxins, inflammation, poor diet, and lack of sleep, it is much harder to experience healing. However, if the path is clear, then healing becomes much easier. Week 1 was about removing the giant boulders from the path. Week 2 is about smoothing the path for quick and effective healing.

Day 8

Day 8 is the start of the process that deals with reducing inflammation and getting into the habit of using essential oils. The body has been cleared of toxins and the essential oils can start to address the general wellbeing of the mind, body, and spirit. Add a few drops of orange and grapefruit oil to a diffuser or the walls of the shower to start the day bright-eyed and bushy-tailed. At midday, add a few drops of black pepper oil to a cotton ball and inhale using the dry evaporation method. Black pepper oil reduces inflammation in the digestive tract and can also have grounding properties. This would be a good time to start practicing creative visualization. Start with a 10-minute session and add an extra 10 minutes of meditation. In the evening, add a few drops of rose and chamomile oil to a warm compress and place on the forehead for 10 minutes before sleeping.

Day 9

Add a few drops of lavender oil to a diffuser while getting ready to start the day. At midday, add a few drops of frankincense oil to a cream and rub onto the hands and temples. Take a few deep breaths with your hands cupped over your nose. Practice a 15-minute detailed creative visualization session and supplement it with a 15-minute workout. In the evening, add a few drops of chamomile oil to a cream or carrier oil and massage into the feet and temples before sleeping.

Day 10

Start the day with a few drops of angelica oil diffused through the room to make sure the body has fully detoxed. At midday, use the dry evaporation method and take a few deep breaths of sandalwood oil. This will help with digestion and has anti-inflammatory properties that can bring balance to the body. In the evening, add a few drops of ylang-ylang and chamomile oil to a warm compress and place on the chest until the compress has lost its heat.

Day 11

Start the day with a 20-minute creative visualization session while diffusing rose and jasmine oil into the space. At midday, add a few drops of ylang-ylang oil to a cream or carrier oil and rub into the temples and hands. In the evening, diffuse lavender, chamomile, and angelica oil into the room before sleeping. Take a break from meditation and exercising as meditation can be challenging for beginners and practicing every day is something that must be learnt. Similarly to bread dough, gluten and elasticity develop better after the dough has been kneaded and left to rest. Periods of work followed by periods of rest can yield the best results.

Day 12

Start the day with a burst of ginger oil to reduce inflammation and improve gut health. At midday, diffuse orange oil into the room to promote focus and engage in a 30-minute meditation session, followed by either a 15-minute creative visualization session or a 20-minute exercise session. In the evening, add a few drops of frankincense and chamomile oil to a warm bath before sleeping.

Day 13

On the penultimate day, make sure the body is adequately detoxed as the final day will be for relaxation and resting. Start the day by adding a few drops of cassia and black pepper oil to a cream or carrier oil and rubbing into the soles of the feet. At midday, diffuse a mixture of grapefruit, orange, and rose oil into the room while engaging in a 30-minute creative visualization session. In the evening, add several drops of chamomile and lavender oil to a linen spray and spray onto the bed before sleeping.

Day 14

Day 14 is about rest and relaxation before the real treatment starts. Bear in mind that not all courses of treatment must follow the same pattern or structure. This guide is merely to show you what is out there, give you some practical experience with essential oils, and prepare the body for healing. Start the day with a mixture of rose, jasmine, and lavender oil. This can be added to a bath or diffused into a room. At midday, practice a 45-minute meditation session while diffusing sandalwood oil into the room. In the evening, add a few drops of chamomile oil to a cream or carrier oil and massage onto the temples, neck, shoulders, and forehead, and thank yourself for your dedication to healing.

This process allows you to try every method of essential oil application while trying and testing a few different oils for different purposes. This 14-day guide will provide you with the necessary information and expertise that you will require on the rest of your journey. Healing will most likely not happen in 14 days. Depending on your situation, relief may be the only possible outcome to look forward to. Either way, starting with a blank slate means that your mind, body, and soul are prepared for the journey to healing. Remember to be patient and kind to yourself on this journey as it won't always be simple or easy. Despite the challenges, essential oils can provide you with the relief you need to move forward.

Conclusion

Contrastingly to the beliefs and practices of modern medicine, healing is about balance. This is why essential oil therapy and aromatherapy are the perfect partners on your journey to healing. Balance is about looking at your being, ailments, pains, fears, successes, and emotions holistically. Instead of separating yourself into three separate and isolated realms, mainly the physical, the emotional, and the spiritual realms, it is important to understand that these realms work together to form one being. Similarly, if you exclusively eat junk food but go to the gym every day, this does not constitute balance. Damage is still being done to your body by filling it with artificial and synthetic foods, whether or not you exercise every day. Balance is not about trying to make up for actions. It is not about binge drinking over the weekend and putting yourself on a detoxifying smoothie cleanse come Monday morning. Balance is about finding equilibrium and moderation in everything you do.

Essential oils probably won't help you with every aspect of your life. They won't change your obnoxious boss into a kind and helpful person. They won't heal your trauma. They won't pay your rent. But essential oil therapy can help you manage the emotional, physical, and spiritual effects of these situations. Sure, your boss may be rude and unhelpful, but changing the way you feel and react to this stimulus can be the difference between falling into a depression and learning from the situation. Essential oils are similar to antidepressants. Antidepressants can drag you out of the darkest pits of a depressive hole, but after that, after you can stand up, you have to begin walking and the antidepressants can't do that for you. To be effective they require some input from you. Similarly, essential oils can help you but only if you help yourself. You do this by living a balanced life. Make sure your diet is balanced, you are getting enough exercise, you practice mindfulness, do things you love, and maintain a positive mindset. It won't always be easy and you might slip and fall occasionally, but healing is never going to be an easy process.

So, why heal—if it's so hard and the journey to healing is so treacherous? One might ask, what is the alternative to healing? First, the alternative is not any easier and leaves you in a bottomless pit of self-pity, misery, unhealthy habits, reclusive tendencies, and depression. None of those things are easy. Healing provides a positive outcome. Healing, while challenging, isn't just a road that leads to nowhere. It leads to happiness, relief, balance, and gratitude. Choosing to heal is choosing to give yourself a fighting chance.

Not sure where to start? To begin, this book is a great resource to have by your side when exploring the world of holistic healing. While it seems basic, it can be easy to treat the symptoms without ever addressing the cause. Essential oils can bring balance to hormones and other aspects of the body, but they may not be able to heal the direct cause. For example, essential oils can ease symptoms of fatigue, but they can't cure menopause. However, in some cases they can heal, for example, if you suffer from insomnia, there are a wide variety of essential oils that you can use to regulate sleeping patterns. As with all holistic healing methods, essential oils won't cure your insomnia if you eat a bunch of sugary food or drink three cups of coffee before bed. This is why holistic healing is challenging, because the level of effectiveness is dependent on you and your actions.

A good way to start is by setting a few goals and being intentional about the process of holistic healing. Start by outlining where you want to go. What is your ultimate goal? Is it to live a healthier lifestyle? Perhaps you want to live a pain-free or happy life? Whatever the goal is, write it down. This is, most likely, a long-term goal. Therefore, to achieve it, you need a set of short-term and medium-term goals. Once you have outlined the ultimate goal, choose two to three medium-term goals to help you reach the long-term goal. This could be anything from exercising three times a week, to meal-prepping, to practicing 30 minutes of meditation every day. Once you have identified the medium-term goals, it is time to set up a few short-term goals to make sure you get started and remain motivated throughout your journey. These goals can be as small as you want them. Actually, they should be very achievable and reachable because you want to make sure you have some successes in your belt before moving on to the more challenging goals. These goals can be anything from exercising for five minutes twice a week, to finishing this book, to cutting down on your intake of sugar for the week. Whatever your goals are, start small. Once you have some confidence, you can up the ante and start to reap the true benefits of essential oil therapy and holistic healing.

Once you have set up your goals and aspirations for the process, it is time to educate yourself on the history of essential oils, the benefits of using essential oils, and ways to incorporate essential oils into your life. This gives you a broader understanding of the process and how you want to progress. Luckily for you, this book has everything you need to know about essential oils as a beginner. If you are ever feeling lost or doubtful, look to the ancient civilizations and religions of this world. Essential oils and plants have been used for millennia and there is no reason why humans should stop anytime soon.

As you move through this journey, you will be able to tailor essential oil therapy and aromatherapy to your own needs. Your understanding of herbs, plants, and spices will burgeon as you enter the world of essential oils and learn how each plant and oil has a specific purpose. Although I have provided a comprehensive list of methods and techniques for using essential oils, there is room for growth and tailoring on your part. If you find that placing a few drops of orange oil, diluted in a carrier oil, on the side of your keyboard makes you feel calmly focused and ready to work, then don't be afraid to do it. Holistic healing is not about following strict and restrictive guidelines. It is about flowing through life in a balanced and intentional way to optimize healing.

Once you have a clear set of goals and a basic understanding of essential oils, it is time to understand how they can help you. Whether you suffer from hair loss, itching, insomnia, fatigue, stress, anxiety, or depression, there is an essential oil that can help you. Remember to always consult a doctor or medical professional because essential oils are not FDA approved or controlled by a regulatory body. Additionally, there are certain essential oils which contradict certain pharmaceutical medications. In this way, make sure essential oils can supplement treatments you may already be using. You don't want to use essential oils to treat one hormonal imbalance just to wake up the next day with a whole new set of hormonal imbalances. While these plants and oils have been used for thousands of years, they are only now being studied clinically and put through rigorous testing. This is why it is important to use essential oils intentionally and in moderation.

It is also crucial to remind yourself of the safety precautions when handling and applying essential oils. Diluting the essential oil before use is quite possibly the most important step in the process of essential oil therapy. If the oil is applied to the skin undiluted, it can cause burns, irritation, dryness, and rashes. The oils extracted from plants are highly concentrated and can have corrosive effects on the skin. However, the opposite is true when purchasing essential oils. If oils are diluted or mixed with any substances other than essential oil, do not purchase it. Would you go into a supermarket and buy juice that has been diluted with water? Probably not because the juice would be bland, and not worth the amount of money you are paying for it. Similarly, some essential oils may seem cheap but that does not mean they are 100% pure. When selecting essential oils, quality is key. Keep in mind which distillation process is used and which plant material has been used. You won't regret spending a little more for a quality product.

Don't be afraid to mix and match, experiment, and use essential oil therapy as a way to let your inner child out. While the symptoms of hormonal imbalance are not pleasant to deal with, the process of healing can be creative, fulfilling, and exciting. Go through some trial and error. While jasmine oil might help you relax, you also might not enjoy the smell of it. There are many other oils to choose from that can help you sleep and satisfy your scent requirements. As I said, holistic healing is not rigid and should be approached flexibly and openly. Most injuries happen when you try to control your body. When you relinquish control and let gravity take you, the chance of injury is lowered (although this mostly applies to survivable situations). Similarly, when starting the journey to holistic healing you must let the process take you where you need to go. Don't try to fight holistic healing with rigid schedules and preconceived notions. Allow yourself to explore the benefits of healing with essential oils.

This is also why practicing mindfulness and meditation can help you *go with the flow*. Being playful and creative is not about mindlessly moving through the process of healing. Playfulness and flexibility take a lot of concentration, work, and intentionality. To be playful, you have to know what works, you have to know your limitations so that you can move within them and work to expand them. Don't just stop using jasmine oil because you don't like the scent. Ask yourself why you don't like the scent. Our brains are very sensitive to smell. It unlocks memories and emotions within our brains that we didn't even know we had. Suddenly you get a whiff of some shoe polish and a flood of images of your dad getting ready for work may enter your mind. Scents and smells have a pervasive influence over the way humans react and function in life. While you might just not like the smell of jasmine, there may be negative connotations lurking behind the facade. If that is the case, you don't need to continue using jasmine oil. Just understanding the emotions and memories behind your aversion to jasmine oil will help you grow and put you on the right track toward holistic healing. Being mindful means living in the present but it also means acting and thinking purposefully. This journey will not only help you to heal your hormonal imbalances or make you feel energized or give you a good night's rest, it will also hold you accountable for your actions, thoughts, and habits. This might feel uncomfortable at first. That is why you must approach the healing process with a sense of acceptance. Accept yourself before the process has even started, before you have had the chance to prove yourself. Accepting and understanding yourself wholeheartedly makes practicing mindfulness less intimidating and more freeing. Self-improvement is not a sign of failure in certain areas, it is a sign of growth. Instead of getting stuck on the things you can't do or the things you need to improve on, use this information to pay respect to the person you once were, and start becoming the person you want to be. The 14-day detox guide is the perfect way to clear the mind, set a few goals, decide what you want for the future, and make it happen. Remember to keep the energy after completing the two-week detox guide. But don't worry about schedules and rigidity. If it does not suit you to meditate and exercise every day, try meditating once a week. The guide is there for you to tip your toes into the world of essential oil therapy. After that, you can adapt the guide to suit your needs, lifestyle, and preferences.

So, before you start your journey to healing, make sure you are invested in yourself and the process. Use this book to guide you through the journey to mental, spiritual, and physical healing as you wander through the chaos of modern civilization. Use essential oils to relieve your symptoms so that you can have the strength to treat the causes. And remember to dilute your oils.

References

Ahuja, N. (2019). Use of essential oils. Ayurveda—Aromatherapy. Ayurveda Awareness Centre. https://www.ayurveda-awareness.com.au/blog/essential-oils-ayurveda-aromatherpy/.

Baker, J. (2020). Hypothyroidism vs. hyperthyroidism: What's the difference? Healthline. https://www.healthline.com/health/hypothyroidism/hypothyroidism-vs-hyperthyroidism.

Ballard, C., O'Brien, J., Reichelt, K., Perry, E. (2002).Aromatherapy as a safe and effective treatment for the management of agitation in severe dementia: the results of a double-blind, placebo-controlled trial with Melissa. *J Clin Psychiatry, 63*(7), 553-558.

Cronkleton, E. (2019). How to use essential oils. Healthline.

https://www.healthline.com/health/how-to-use-essential-oils.

Elbanhnasawy, A. (2019). The impact or thyme and rosemary on prevention of osteoporosis in rats. *Journal of Nutrition and Metabolism.*

Enshaieh, S., Jooya, A., Siadat, A., Iraji, F. (2007). The efficacy of 5% topical tea tree oil gel in mild to moderate acne vulgaris: a randomized, double-blind placebo-controlled study. *Indian J Dermatol Venereol Leprol, 73*(1), 22-25.

FGB Natural Products. (N.d.). History of essential oils.

https://www.fgb.com.au/content/history-essential-oils.

Fisher, K., Phillips, C. (2006). The effect of lemon, orange and bergamot essential oils and their components on the survival of Campylobacter jejuni, Escherichia coli O157, Listeria monocytogenes, Bacillus cereus and Staphylococcus aureus in vitro and in food systems. *The Journal of Microbiology, 101*(6), 1232-1240.

Hafner, C. (N.d.). Five phases of transformation or the five elements. University of Minnesota. https://www.takingcharge.csh.umn.edu/expl ore-healing-practices/what-traditional-chinese-medicine/what-qi-and-other-concepts/five-phases-t

Halcon, L. (N.d.). What are essential oils? University of Minnesota. https://www.takingcharge.csh.umn.edu/wha t-are-essential-oils.

Hay, I., Jamieson, M., Ormerod, A. (1998). Randomized trial of aromatherapy. Successful treatment for alopecia areata. *Arch Dermatol, 134*(11), 1349-1352.

Huizen, J. (2020). What to know about hormonal imbalances.

Medical News Today. https://www.medicalnewstoday.com/articles/321486.

International Federation of Aromatherapists. (N.d.) History of aromatherapy. https://ifaroma.org/en_GB/home/explore_aromatherapy/about-aromatherapy/history-aromatherapy.

Mizrahi, B., Shapira, L., Domb, A., Houri-Haddad, Y. (2006). Citrus oil and MgCl2 as antibacterial and anti-inflammatory agents. *J Periodontol, 77*(6), 963-968.

New Directions Aromatics. (2017). Uncapping the power of nature: Essential oil extraction methods. https://www.newdirectionsaromatics.com/blog/articles/how-essential-oils-are-made.html.

Newton, I. (N.d.). Isaac Newton quotes. Brainy Quote. https://www.brainyquote.com/authors/isaac-newton-quotes

Pick, M. (2018). 7 great essential oils for balancing hormones. Marcelle Pick. https://marcellepick.com/7-essential-oils-for-hormones/.

Stierwalt, S. (2019). Do essential oils work? Here's what science says. Quick and dirty tips. https://www.quickanddirtytips.com/education/science/do-essential-oils-work-heres-what-science-says.

Suhr, K., I., Nielsen, P., V. (2003). Antifungal activity of essential oils evaluated by two different application techniques against rye bread spoilage fungi. *Journal of Applied Microbiology, 94*, 665-674.

Taiji Forum. (N.d.). Basics of Tai Chi. https://taiji-forum.com/tai-chi-taiji/basics/.

WebMD. (2019). Dos and don'ts of essential oils. https://www.webmd.com/skin-problems-and-treatments/ss/slideshow-essential-oils.

West, H. (2019). What are essential oils, and do they work? Healthline. https://www.healthline.com/nutrition/what-are-essential-oils#bottom-line.

Your Hormones. (N.d.). Glands. You and your hormones. https://www.yourhormones.info/glands/.

www.ingramcontent.com/pod-product-compliance
Lightning Source LLC
Chambersburg PA
CBHW070924030426
42336CB00014BA/2524